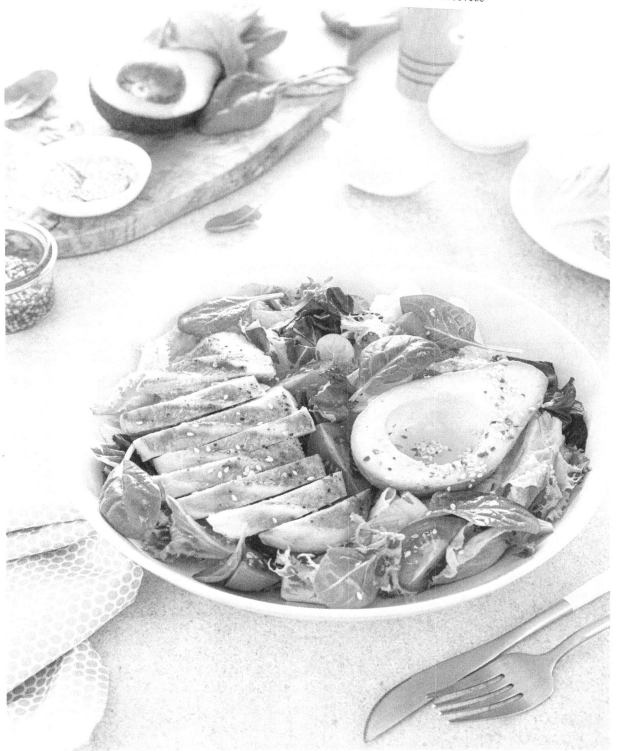

THE DR. NOWZARADAN

BIBLE

6 IN 1

Get Ready to Live a Better, Healthy and Enjoyable Life | Lose up to 30 Pounds with 1200-Calorie Affordable Recipes and Meal Plans Suitable For Every Age

Nathalie Kimmel

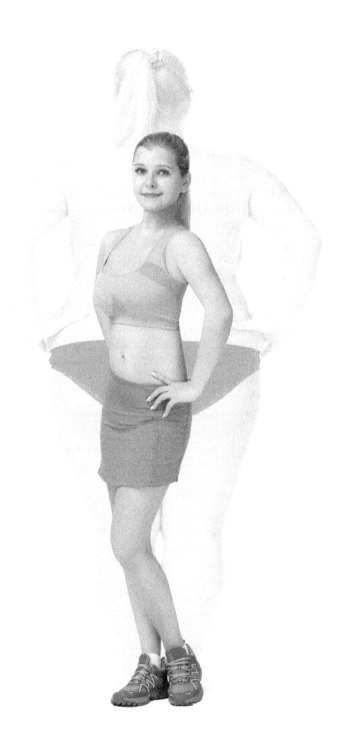

Table of Contents

BOOK 1:   WHO IS DR. NOWZARADAN 7

  INTRODUCTION 8
  CHAPTER 1.   DR. YOUNAN NOWZARADAN 10

BOOK 2:   SECRETS OF DR. NOWZARADAN'S DIET PLAN 13

  INTRODUCTION 14
  CHAPTER 1.   HOW TO START THE DIET 15
  CHAPTER 2.   BASIC BENEFITS AND SUCCESS SECRETS OF THE DIET ... 17
    Benefits of Dr. Now's Diet 18
    Downsides of Dr. Now's Diet 18
  CHAPTER 3.   DISEASES THAT THE DIET COMBATS 20
    The Importance of Pre-Surgery Weight Loss 21
    Weight Loss Tips 21
  CHAPTER 4.   TRICKS AND TIPS TO NOT STOP THE DIET 22
    Things to Keep in Mind 23

BOOK 3:   DR. NOWZARADAN'S DIET PLAN FOR BEGINNERS 25

  INTRODUCTION 26
  CHAPTER 1.   BREAKFAST 28
    Apple Pancakes 28
    Baked Beans 29
    Roasted Root Vegetable Hash 30
    Turkey Caprese Meatloaf Cups 31
    Veggie Omelet 32
  CHAPTER 2.   LUNCH 33
    Balsamic Chicken and Beans 33
    Lavender Lamb Chops 34
    Paprika and Feta Cheese on Chicken Skillet 35
    Spicy Chicken Leg Quarters 36
    Trout and Endives 37
  CHAPTER 3.   DINNER 38
    Chicken and Mushrooms 38
    Hot Turkey Meatballs 39
    Pasta with Alfredo Sauce 40
    Seared Haddocks with Beets 41
    Turkey Artichokes 42
  CHAPTER 4.   SNACKS 43
    Fiery Shrimp Cocktail Salad 43
    Honey Granola 44
    Pesto Veggie Pinwheels 45
    Spinach Chips with Avocado Hummus 46
    Sweet Butternut 47
  CHAPTER 5.   SOUPS AND SIDE DISHES 48

Butternut Squash Soup 48

Classic Tabbouleh 49

Crispy Herb Cauliflower Florets 50

White Bean Soup 51

Wonton Soup 52

CHAPTER 6.   30-DAY MEAL PLAN 53

BOOK 4:   DR. NOWZARADAN'S MEAL PLAN ON A BUDGET 55

INTRODUCTION 56

CHAPTER 1.   BREAKFAST 58

Brussels Sprouts Delight 58

Cauliflower Based Waffles 59

Eggs and Veggies 60

Spiced Oatmeal 61

Zucchini Skilletcakes 62

CHAPTER 2.   LUNCH 63

Cashew Chicken Curry 63

Honey Balsamic Salmon and Lemon Asparagus 64

Miso Chicken with Sesame 65

Spaghetti Bolognese 66

Veal Parmesan 67

CHAPTER 3.   DINNER 68

Bell Peppers and Sausage 68

Brown Rice Pilaf with Butternut Squash 69

Green Bean Casserole 70

Nut-Crusted Chicken Breasts 71

Tangy Chicken Drumsticks 72

CHAPTER 4.   SNACKS 73

Avocado Tuna Bites 73

Chicken Salad with Parmesan 74

Creamed Peas 75

Mushroom Sausages 76

White Cabbage and Lentils with Relish 77

CHAPTER 5.   SOUPS AND SIDE DISHES 78

Basil Zucchini Soup 78

Ham and Bean Soup 79

Paprika and Chives Potatoes 80

Pesto Broccoli Quinoa 81

Vegetable Panini 82

CHAPTER 6.   30-DAY MEAL PLAN 83

BOOK 5:   DR. NOWZARADAN'S LOW CARB HIGH PROTEIN RECIPES 85

INTRODUCTION 86

CHAPTER 1.   BREAKFAST 88

Chicken Souvlaki 88

Eggs Florentine 89

Ground Pork Wonton Ravioli 90

Onion Frittata 91

Veggie Quiche Muffins 92

CHAPTER 2.   LUNCH **93**

Chicken Calzone 93

Chicken Cordon Bleu 94

Crispy Pollock and Gazpacho 95

Thyme Ginger Garlic Beef 96

Zucchini and Lemon Herb Salmon 97

CHAPTER 3.   DINNER **98**

Asparagus and Lemon Salmon 98

Balsamic Steaks 99

Crab Mushrooms 100

Seared Scallops and Roasted Grapes 101

Turnip Greens and Artichoke Chicken 102

CHAPTER 4.   SNACKS **103**

Cinnamon Stuffed Peaches 103

Mashed Beets 104

Pork Beef Bean Nachos 105

Shrimps Ceviche 106

Spiced Tea Pudding 107

CHAPTER 5.   SOUP AND SIDE DISHES **108**

Coconut and Lemongrass Turkey Soup 108

Margherita Slices 109

Smoked Salmon, Avocado, and Cucumber Bites 110

Spicy Carrot and Lime Soup 111

White Bean and Kale Soup with Chicken 112

CHAPTER 6.   30-DAY MEAL PLAN **113**

BOOK 6:   BONUS: LOW-CALORIE KETO RECIPES **115**

INTRODUCTION **116**

CHAPTER 1.   THE KETO DIET **118**

CHAPTER 2.   KETO RECIPES **121**

Baked Granola 121

Beef with Kale and Leeks 122

Hot Dog Rolls 123

Lamb with Fennel and Figs 124

Pork Schnitzel 125

Ricotta Cloud Pancakes with Whipped Cream 126

Sausage Egg Cups 127

Shrimp and Olives Pan 128

Shrimp Risotto 129

Veal Picatta 130

BOOK 1.
WHO IS DR. NOWZARADAN

Introduction

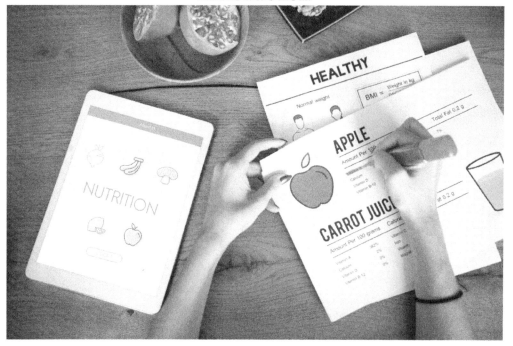

There is more to losing weight than finding a surgeon, being approved for surgery, and, finally, having the procedure. For many, developing positive habits and breaking away from destructive old habits can be very challenging. You will need to cope with stress and daily struggles without reaching for food, but making these changes does get easier over time.

If you've never exercised before, you may be pleasantly surprised to find that you enjoy the activity and the stress relief that comes along with it. Taking an hour a day out of your busy life to exercise may provide multiple benefits.

Finding support from friends, family, and even fellow weight loss surgery patients will be instrumental in your success. Finding someone willing to listen or someone who understands what you are going through is an invaluable part of the process.

It is safe to say that your life will be dramatically different after your surgery, mostly in very positive ways. As your body shrinks, you will feel better, look better, have more energy, and be a much healthier person than you ever imagined. If you doubt how much better you will feel after your weight loss, pick up a sack of potatoes at the grocery store the next time you are shopping and see how long it takes before your arms get tired. You will be losing that weight many times, and no longer carrying those extra pounds with every step will feel fantastic.

Fitting into smaller sizes, improving your self-confidence, and going up a flight of stairs or out for a walk without being exhausted will be just a few of the rewards of your weight loss. While weight loss surgery isn't going to make all of your troubles go away, it may make health problems such as high blood pressure, sleep apnea, and type 2 diabetes disappear.

Things you may have avoided in the past will become far more accessible as you lose weight. Imagine going to a movie and fitting comfortably into the movie seat or taking a vacation to a sunny beach and wearing a bathing suit without feeling self-conscious. As you work toward your weight loss goal, you will be meeting other purposes, such as being able to run and play with your children or walking from one actual end of the mall to the other without a second thought.

Chapter 1.
Dr. Younan Nowzaradan

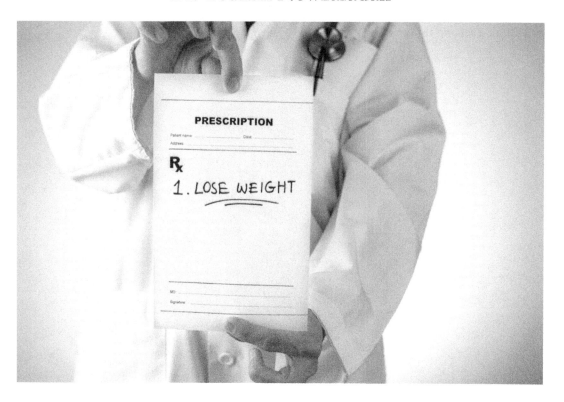

Dr. Younan Nowzaradan, who is renowned for performing surgery on patients who are obese on the TLC reality program "My 600-Lb. Life," is the brains behind the Dr. Now Diet, which is a very stringent low-calorie and low-carbohydrate eating plan. The Dr. Now Diet was designed by Nowzaradan. Patients who weigh more than 600 pounds before weight-loss surgery are followed by the program both before and after the procedure.

In order to better prepare patients for bariatric surgery, Nowzaradan recommends that patients follow the diet prescribed by Dr. Now. Nowzaradan is the author of the book "The Scale Does Not Lie, People Do," which was published in 2013.

Bariatric Surgery

- Gastric bypass. The Roux-en-Y gastric bypass, which is more often referred to as just gastric bypass, will make your stomach smaller. Surgeons will use the upper portion of your stomach to construct a tiny pouch in your abdomen. As part of the bypass procedure, a little section of your small intestine, known as the jejunum, will be connected to a hole in this new pouch. This will enable food to move directly from the pouch to your small intestine. Because of this, the quantity of food that you are able to ingest is decreased, and you are able to take in less calories as a result.

- Sleeve gastrectomy. When you have this particular operation, about three quarters of your stomach will be removed. What is left is a segment that is either in the form of a tube or a sleeve, and it can only hold a small portion of the food it once did. According to Dr. Xiaoxi Feng, a bariatric surgeon at the Cleveland Clinic in Ohio, the effects of this treatment are irreversible.

- Duodenal switch. A duodenal switch reduces the amount of food that is absorbed by the stomach. This method, which is more formally called as biliopancreatic diversion with duodenal switch, is a hybrid procedure that combines aspects of sleeve gastrectomy and bypass. According to Feng, bariatric surgeons perform a more comprehensive version of gastric bypass surgery during the duodenal switch operation.

- Lap-band. Laparoscopic gastric banding, also known as an adjustable gastric band, is a treatment that involves the implantation of a soft implant that incorporates an expanding balloon around the top of your stomach. This technique is also known as an adjustable gastric band. This causes the stomach to be divided into two portions, and you are only able to consume enough food to fill the upper segment.

Dr. Erik P. Dutson, surgical director of the Center for Obesity and Metabolic Health at UCLA in Westwood, California, says bariatric surgeons and patients examine several aspects before choosing an option.

"Most U.S. bariatric surgery clinics do either gastric bypass or sleeve gastrectomy," he explains. "Most patients will perform well with either procedure, but others should not receive one due to medical issues. Larger individuals, those with advanced diabetes, and those with GERD (a disease in which stomach contents flow back up via the lower esophageal sphincter) perform better with gastric bypass."

Sleeve gastrectomy helps people with immunological suppression (such as organ transplant patients).

Dr. Judy Chen-Meekin, a surgeon and bariatric expert at the University of Washington School of Medicine, believes patients should be comfortable with the surgical choice, but medical factors typically drive the decision.

Measurement Conversions

Volume Equivalents (Dry)

US STANDARD	METRIC (APPROXIMATE)
⅛ teaspoon	0.5 mL
¼ teaspoon	1 mL
½ teaspoon	2 mL
¾ teaspoon	4 mL
1 teaspoon	5 mL
1 tablespoon	15 mL
¼ cup	59 mL
⅓ cup	79 mL
½ cup	118 mL
⅔ cup	156 mL
¾ cup	177 mL
1 cup	235 mL
2 cups or 1 pint	475 mL
3 cups	700 mL
4 cups or 1 quart	1 L
½ gallon	2 L
1 gallon	4 L

Volume Equivalents (Liquid)

US STANDARD	US STANDARD (OUNCES)	METRIC (APPROXIMATE)
2 tablespoons	1 fl. oz.	30 mL
¼ cup	2 fl. oz.	60 mL
½ cup	4 fl. oz.	120 mL
1 cup	8 fl. oz.	240 mL
1½ cups	12 fl. oz.	355 mL
2 cups or 1 pint	16 fl. oz.	475 mL
4 cups or 1 quart	32 fl. oz.	1 L
1 gallon	128 fl. oz.	4 L

Oven Temperatures

FAHRENHEIT (F)	CELSIUS (C) (APPROXIMATE)
250°F	120°C
300°F	150°C
325°F	165°C
350°F	180°C
375°F	190°C
400°F	200°C
425°F	220°C
450°F	230°C

BOOK 2.
SECRETS OF DR. NOWZARADAN'S DIET PLAN

Introduction

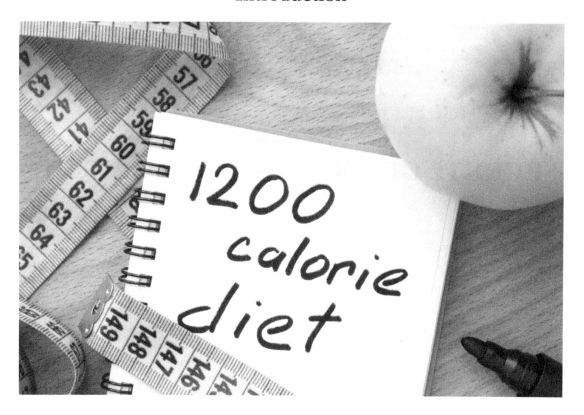

Dr. Nowzaradan's diet involves sticking to a 1,200-calorie-per-day diet. The strategy emphasizes maintaining a well-balanced diet while lowering your calorie intake. It is possible to lose weight easily by adopting Dr. Now's diet.

This diet plan is low in calories and focuses on eating foods that are low in carbs and fat, high in protein and vitamins, and helping your body get the nutrients it needs to stay healthy.

Dr. Now's diet plan approach includes sticking to a strict 1,200-calorie (maximum) diet schedule. Some of the more serious, morbidly obese patients set their calorie limit as low as 1,000 calories. The main idea of the diet is to cut calorie consumption to approximately 1,200 calories daily without eliminating any essential foods except sugar.

This strict diet consists of a mix of low-fat, low-carb, and high-protein foods. The majority of the diet plan seems to be promising: eating a lot of plant-based proteins, staying hydrated, and keeping track of eating habits. The drawback is the lengthy list of foods that must be avoided.

Chapter 1.
How to Start the Diet

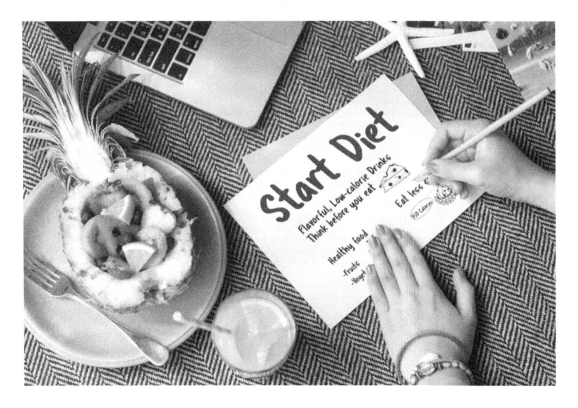

Whether you have been overweight for years or you just recently discovered that you are, you may want to consider changing your lifestyle.

1. Get more sleep

Not getting enough sleep can lead to increased risk for heart disease, high blood pressure, obesity and type 2 diabetes. You also need to limit your naps. Try to get exercise during the day, but avoid exercising within two hours before you go to bed.

2. Start an exercise routine

Begin by staying active during the day. If you are already physically active, try to challenge yourself by beginning an exercise routine. When you do decide to start an exercise routine, find an exercise that you like.

3. Detoxify your body

Detoxifying your body can help reduce the risk of developing food-related illnesses and weight gain.

For example, you can have white meat instead of red meat, turkey instead of chicken, and regular pasta instead of wheat pasta.

The Dr. Now Diet can also be supplemented with vitamin and mineral supplements.

4. Take better care of yourself

You can also improve your lifestyle by taking better care of yourself. Start by getting enough sleep, exercising, and eating healthier foods.

Chapter 2
Basic Benefits and Success Secrets of the Diet

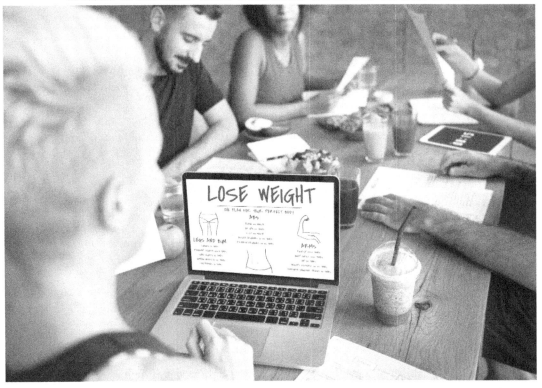

Weight loss is one of the main advantages of Dr. Now's diet. When the calorie intake is limited, the body burns accumulated fat to maintain proper operation. What follows is a rapid weight loss. As a result, you get much better sleep, avoid the risk of knee pain or high blood pressure.

This strict, low calorie diet plan does result in fast weight loss, especially in people with higher body weight. Dr. Now encourages many of his patients who weigh more than 600 pounds (272 kg) to try to lose 30 pounds (14 kg) in just 30 days, and many of them are successful.

In fact, the 1,200 calorie diet is commonly used for preoperative bariatric surgery patients, not just in Dr. Now's practice.

In one study on 24 women with obesity, participants lost a significant amount of weight with and without exercise in just 13 days. Doctors often recommend preoperative weight loss for people undergoing bariatric surgery because it appears to help reduce complications after the operation. One study looked at outcomes in more than 480,000 people who had bariatric surgery. The researchers found that weight loss prior to surgery helped reduce the risk of death within 30 days of surgery — even when people lost less than 5% of their body weight.

Studies have also found that when people were required to lose weight before they were approved to have weight loss surgery, they tended to have more successful weight outcomes after surgery.

The Dr. Now Diet can induce rapid weight loss, and preoperative weight loss does appear to help improve outcomes in people who have weight loss surgery.

Benefits of Dr. Now's Diet

The main benefit of the Dr. Now diet is that it's very effective for fast weight loss.

However, there isn't anything special about the diet for weight loss perse, other than it's low in calories.

Keep in mind that weight loss only occurs when you consume fewer calories than you need to support normal bodily functions and any physical activity.

The greater the calorie deficit, the more weight you will lose over a shorter period.

The patients to whom Dr. Now prescribes his diet plan may need anywhere from 3,000 to 4,000 calories per day just to maintain their weight.

As you can imagine, putting the patients on a 1,000-1,200 calorie diet will result in rapid weight loss due to the large calorie deficit.

But even if the number of calories you need to maintain your weight is not as high as the patients on "My 600-lb. Life," the 1,000-1,200 calories that the diet allows is well below most people's calorie needs.

Downsides of Dr. Now's Diet

While effective for rapid weight loss, the diet has several downsides.

The main disadvantage is that it can be difficult to follow long-term due to the diet's rigidity and potential side effects.

So even though the diet is effective for weight loss, if you can't follow the diet for very long, it's useless.

Common side effects associated with a low-calorie diet like Dr. Now's include:

- constant hunger
- low energy
- low sex drive
- irritability

- poor sleep quality

- constipation

- headaches

- dizziness

- hair thinning

- amenorrhea

- cold intolerance

Although these side effects are minor, they can significantly interfere with your work or school performance as well as your relationships with family and friends.

The diet is also likely lacking in certain vitamins and minerals, like magnesium, vitamin D, calcium, thiamin, and potassium (2).

While short-term nutrient shortfalls are unlikely to pose any immediate health risks, following the diet for several weeks to months could lead to health problems.

Chapter 3
Diseases That the Diet Combats

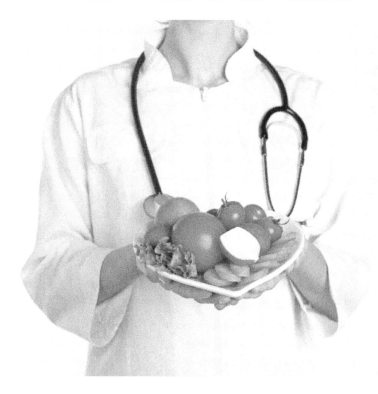

Unless you are morbidly obese and considering lap band system surgery or similar drastic measures, I don't think the Dr. Nowzardan eating plan would be right for you.

That said, you can pick up some valuable tips to apply to your healthy lifestyle plan. Prime examples of easy and noticeable changes to make would be using greek yogurt instead of sweetened because eliminating sugar can help wean you off junk food cravings.

He also has a flat ban on potatoes because it acts almost like a trigger for the more problematic foods or behaviors. This is a strict diet, but it's also important to note that it is highly individualized and tailored to each dieter.

This is why you can't find hard guidelines for the eating plan online. Because it isn't a one glove fits all type deal, the only way you could get a similar program is through a nutritionist of your own.

The Importance of Pre-Surgery Weight Loss

Surgery always comes with an inherent risk. This risk is much higher when the patient is morbidly obese. Dr. Now's 1200 calorie diet is designed as both proofs of the patient's commitment to turning their life around and every pound shed on the diet lessening their risk on the operating table.

The 1200 calories diet is a high protein focusing on portion control and eating whole and natural foods.

This is owing to Dr. Now's belief that a lot of obesity is due to the pre-packaged processed foods prevalent in the modern supermarket.

Weight Loss Tips

Dr. Now's diet recommends losing weight by trying to eliminate snacking from your daily routine. Research has shown that eating frequently can lead to high blood sugar content and weight retained around the waist.

By focusing on three square meals with appropriate portion control, the 1200 calories diet builds habits to keep the weight off.

1200 calories are significantly less than what most people are used to eating in a day. This deficit proves dedication to weight loss and a strong base for losing weight before the surgery. The diet plan is made possible by the recommended meals' high protein content helping patients feel fuller for longer.

Chapter 4
Tricks and Tips to not Stop the Diet

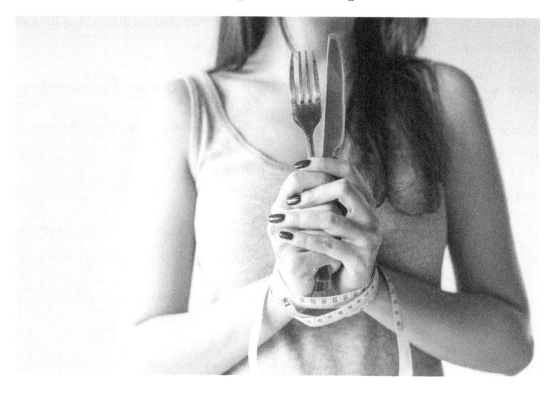

There are no taget in the 1200 diet plan. The basic strategy is straightforward and straightforward. Your entire caloric consumption must be less than or equal to 1,200 calories per day in order to stay within the diet plan's restrictions. Muffin Top, Lose It, Cron-o-meter, FatSecret, and SparkPeople are just a few of the apps that may help you actually keep track of how many calories you eat.

Because the diet is more essential for weight loss than for weight maintenance, it is critical that you set a weight goal for yourself and take care to avoid losing muscle mass when losing weight. You have the option of raising your calorie intake after you have reached your goal weight; nevertheless, you should maintain your healthy eating habits to keep your weight under control.

It is my responsibility to advise you that if you choose to follow this diet, you will likely consume less calories per day than you may think if you are accustomed to eating a lot of calories. This is due to the fact that your body may be compelled to feel hunger while taking the supplement.

To counteract the sensations of hunger that are prevalent while dieting, it is important to eat meals that are both healthy and will keep you feeling full for a long amount of time. Eat a little quantity of healthy and satiating meals to satisfy your appetite.

Watermelon, salad, grapefruit, vegetables, fruits with a high water content, and other healthy meals are just a few of the numerous possibilities available.

The plan allows you to have snacks in between each of your three meals, as well as eating six times per day with snacks in between those meals. It will also allow you to participate in less intense activity, which will help you attain your weight reduction goal. On a salors deficit, rgorou exercise may be detrimental.

Check to determine whether your 1200 calorie meal plan includes a healthy and well-balanced selection of meals when following this diet plan. This is necessary to ensure that you do not have any nutritional deficiencies and that you drink enough water on a regular basis to stay hydrated and maintain good hunger control.

Things to Keep in Mind

Cereals: Whole wheat, millet, ragi, amaranth, oats, and barley are high-fiber, multi-nutrient grains to include in your diet. Use these different flours to add diversity to your meals. Breakfast would be better served with a bowl of multigrain cereal rather than refined, sugar-coated, rose-flavored cereal. It doesn't mean you shouldn't eat refined grains; rather, it implies you should only do so on rare occasions. Polished rice, which includes Idlu, Doa, and Uttaram, is one refined grain that is ideal for picking as a healthy diet alternative. To prepare a high-fiber salad, replace it for arugula and top white bread with a significant number of raw veggies.

These are essential for our bodies' growth, repair, and maintenance, as well as our hormones, blood, and immune systems. Eating meals with at least one type of protein may help you consume less cereal. Dal, besan, ou, raneer, and shee are all examples of vegetable sources of protein. Choose lower calorie alternatives to paneer and cheese, which are both rich in fat calories. In compared to beef, organ meats, and pig, chicken, fish, and eggs are the healthiest non-vegetarian protein sources, in that order.

Fat: You can control how many calories you consume by controlling how much you eat, and you can do so without sacrificing taste or losing any of the health advantages that come with it. Even while refined vegetable oils are healthful, you should not restrict yourself to just one kind. Ghee and clarified butter contain the same amount of calories and fat as vegetable oil, however clarified butter and ghee have a greater saturated fat content. 1tr/dau is ok.

Vegetables: Finally, a cuisine that will satiate your hunger to the utmost degree possible. Hungry? For a warm and salty snack, eat a carrot, boil your veggies, combine them, and create a soup out of them, or juice your vegetables for a cold and refreshing drink. 3 serving each day is recommended. A leafy vegetable serving weighs 150 grams, whereas any other vegetable serving weighs 100 grams. However, you have no need to be concerned about your weight since you are free to eat as much as you want. The satsh onlu is reserved for root and tuber delicacies like rotato, sweet rotato, uam, and others. They are actually and really capable of providing you with the same amount of calories as their part of a meal.

Fruit: These create a delicious dessert. Take two servings of 100-150 grams each of banana and mango (when in season). Milk and milk-based products Each meal should include some kind of milk, such as skim milk, fat-free dahi, or skim milk ricotta. You might also use ricotta made from skim milk. In fact, a late-night need for anything sweet may be satisfied with a fat-free milk ruddling. Regardless of how many calories you wish to eat, be sure you are not depriving yourself of the taste of food in any manner. Eat seasonally, try new cuisines, and consume your meals in their whole. Maintaining your health will not actually and only help you maintain your present weight, but will also give you a radiant complexion and lots of energy.

BOOK 3.
DR. NOWZARADAN'S DIET PLAN FOR BEGINNERS

Introduction

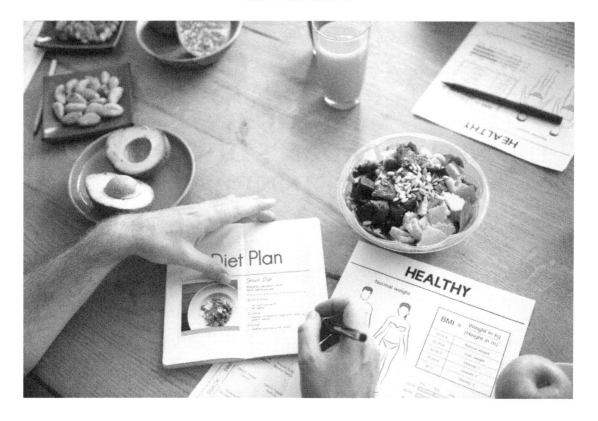

If you're a fan of the show like me, you know that Dr. Now prescribes a 1,000–1,200 calorie diet plan — referred to as the Dr. Now diet — for his patients before performing weight loss surgery.

If you're a fan of the show like me, you know that Dr. Now prescribes a 1,000–1,200 calorie diet plan — referred to as the Dr. Now diet — for his patients before performing weight loss surgery. Although this diet plan can be followed by, anyone, it is best suited for overweight or obese people who want to lose weight. The Dr. Now fascinating career contains an unique route to protect health, increase exercise chances, and, ultimately, lose weight.

The primary concept of Dr. Now's diet plan is to reduce calorie intake to about 1200 calories a day, without excluding any food groups, except sugar.

The diet encourages patients to reduce calorie intake and eat a healthy balanced diet. This helps them lose weight, the healthy way. In preparation from the show, Dr. Now has an ample diet and exercise recipes that can be followed to help people lose weight.

One of the good things about Dr. Now's 1200 calorie diet is that food is the only indicator of calorie intake that is important according to Dr. Now. You can eat any food you want, if it has 1200 calories or less. But, if you choose to complete Dr.Now's 1200 calorie diet if you choose, you must make certain it is a healthy weight loss plan. However, if you're looking to lose weight, you may wonder whether the diet can work for you. Eating 1200 calories a day is the lowest level that will work for your body. It is higher than one recommended by many dietcrafters as a first step in a weight loss plan.

Chapter 1.
Breakfast

Apple Pancakes

Serving Size: 8

Cooking Time: 9 minutes

Ingredients:

- ¼ cup of extra-virgin olive oil, divided
- 1 cup of whole wheat flour
- 2 teaspoons of baking powder
- 1 teaspoon of baking soda
- 1 teaspoon of ground cinnamon
- 1 cup of 1% milk
- 2 large eggs
- 1 medium Gala apple, diced
- 2 tablespoons of maple syrup
- ¼ cup of chopped walnuts

Directions:

- Set aside 1 teaspoon of oil to use for oiling a griddle or skillet. Mix the eggs, baking soda, apple, baking powder, milk, cinnamon.
- Oil and heat the pan, pour in about ¼ cup of the batter for each pancake. Cook until browned on both sides.
- To serve, drizzle each serving with 1 tablespoon of walnuts and drizzle with ½ tablespoon of maple syrup.

Nutritional Values: Calories 378; Carbs 39g; Fat 22g; Protein 10g

Baked Beans

Serving Size: 8

Cooking Time: 4 hours 20 minutes

Ingredients:

- ¾ cup of dry pinto beans
- ¾ cup of dry red kidney beans
- ¾ cup of dry navy beans
- 5 cups of low-sodium vegetable stock
- 1 medium onion peeled and halved
- 1/3 cup of molasses
- 1 tablespoon of Dijon mustard
- 1 teaspoon of salt
- ½ cup of chopped canned tomatoes
- 1 tablespoon of apple cider vinegar

Directions:

- Soak beans overnight after picking and sorting.
- Preheat oven to 250°F.
- Drain beans and place in a large-sized pot with vegetable stock, then bring to a boil over high heat and simmer for 30 minutes.
- Place beans in a 2 ½ quart baking dish with onion.
- Mix remaining ingredients. Pour over beans, covering them completely, then cover dish and bake for 4 hours, checking every ½ hour and adding more reserved stock if needed.

Nutritional Values: Calories 250; Carbs 49g; Fat 1g; Protein 13g

Roasted Root Vegetable Hash

Serving Size: 4

Cooking Time: 40 minutes

Ingredients:

- Cooking spray
- 2 small sweet potatoes, peeled and cubed
- 2 parsnips, peeled and sliced
- 1 red onion, thinly sliced
- 2 tablespoons olive oil
- ½ tablespoon balsamic vinegar
- ¼ teaspoon kosher or sea salt
- ½ teaspoon ground black pepper
- ¼ teaspoon crushed red pepper flakes
- 8 Perfectly Poached Eggs

Directions:

- Preheat the oven to 400°F. Brush baking sheet with the cooking spray.
- Place the sweet potatoes, parsnips, and red onion on the greased baking sheet. Pour the prepared olive oil and balsamic vinegar and season with the salt, black pepper, and crushed red pepper flakes. Toss to coat.
- Roast for 35 to 40 minutes, until vegetables are fork tender and crispy on the outside.
- Serve with Perfectly Poached Eggs.
- Evenly divide the hash and eggs into microwaveable airtight containers. Heat it again in the microwave on high for 1 to 2 minutes.

Nutritional Values: Calories 343; Carbs 33g; Fat 17g; Protein 15g

Turkey Caprese Meatloaf Cups

Serving Size: 6

Cooking Time: 35 minutes

Ingredients:

- 1 large egg
- 2 pounds ground turkey breast
- 3 pieces of sun-dried tomatoes,
- Drained and chopped
- ¼ cup fresh basil leaves, chopped
- 5 ounces low-fat fresh mozzarella, shredded
- ½ teaspoon garlic powder
- ¼ teaspoon salt and ½ teaspoon pepper, to taste

Directions:

- Preheat oven to 400°F.
- Beat the egg in a big mixing container.
- Add the remaining ingredients and mix everything with your hands until evenly combined.
- Spray a 12-cup muffin tin and divide the turkey mixture among the muffin cups, pressing the mix in. Cook in the preheated oven till the turkey is well-cooked for about 25-30 minutes.
- Chill the meatloaves entirely and store them in a container in the fridge for up to 5 days.

Nutritional Values: Calories 181; Carbs 4g; Fat 11g; Protein 43g

Veggie Omelet

Serving Size: 3

Cooking Time: 20 minutes

Ingredients:

- 3 egg whites
- 1 egg
- 1/2 teaspoon extra-virgin olive oil
- 1/8 teaspoon red pepper flakes
- 1/8 teaspoon ground nutmeg
- 1/8 teaspoon garlic powder
- A Pinch of salt
- 1/8 teaspoon ground black pepper
- 1/2 cup sliced fresh mushrooms
- 2 tablespoons chopped red bell pepper
- 1/4 cup chopped green onion
- 1/2 cup chopped tomato
- 1 cup chopped fresh spinach

Directions:

- In a large-sized bowl, whisk together egg whites, egg, garlic powder, red pepper flakes, nutmeg, salt and pepper until well blended.
- Heat olive oil in a prepared large-sized skillet over medium heat; add green onion, mushrooms and belle pepper and cook for approximately about 5 minutes or until tender; stir in tomato and egg mixture and cook for approximately about 5 minutes per side or until egg is set. Slice and serve hot.

Nutritional Values: Calories 286; Carbs 31g; Fat 11.5g; Protein 10.9g

Chapter 2.
Lunch

Balsamic Chicken and Beans

Serving Size: 4

Cooking Time: 40 minutes

Ingredients:

- 1 lb. trimmed fresh green beans
- ¼ c. balsamic vinegar
- 2 sliced shallots
- 2 tablespoons Red pepper flakes
- 4 skinless, de-boned chicken breasts
- 2 minced garlic cloves
- 3 tablespoons Extra virgin olive oil

Directions:

- Combine 2 tablespoons of the prepared olive oil with the balsamic vinegar, garlic, and shallots. Pour it over the chicken breasts and refrigerate overnight.
- The next day, preheat the oven to 375 0F.
- Take the chicken out of the marinade and arrange in a shallow baking pan. Discard the rest of the marinade.
- Bake in the oven for 40 minutes.
- While the chicken is actually cooking, bring a large pot of water to a boil.
- Place the green beans in the water and allow them to cook for five minutes and then drain.
- Heat one tablespoon of olive oil in the pot and return the green beans after rinsing them.
- Toss with red pepper flakes.

Nutritional Values: Calories 433; Fat 17.4g; Carbohydrates 12.9g; Protein 56.1g

Lavender Lamb Chops

Serving Size: 4

Cooking Time: 25 minutes

Ingredients:

- 2 tablespoons rosemary, chopped
- 1 and ½ pounds lamb chops
- Salt and black pepper to the taste
- 1 tablespoon lavender, chopped
- 2 garlic cloves, minced
- 3 red oranges, cut in halves
- 2 small pieces of orange peel
- A drizzle of olive oil
- 1 teaspoon ghee

Directions:

- In a large-sized bowl, mix lamb chops with salt, pepper, rosemary, lavender, garlic and orange peel, toss to coat and leave aside for a couple of hours.
- Grease your kitchen grill with ghee, heat up over medium high heat, place lamb chops on it, cook for 3 minutes, flip, squeeze 1 orange half over them, cook for 3 minutes more, flip them again, cook them for 2 minutes and squeeze another orange half over them.
- Place lamb chops on a plate and keep them warm for now..
- Add remaining orange halves on preheated grill, cook them for 3 minutes, flip and cook them for another 3 minutes.
- Divide lamb chops on plates, add orange halves on the side, drizzle some olive oil over them and serve.
- Enjoy!

Nutritional Values: Calories 250; Carbs 5g; Fat 5g; Protein 8g

Paprika and Feta Cheese on Chicken Skillet

Serving Size: 3

Cooking Time: 30 minutes

Ingredients:

- ¼ cup black olives, sliced in circles
- ½ teaspoon coriander
- ½ teaspoon paprika
- 1 ½ cups diced tomatoes with the juice
- 1 cup yellow onion, chopped
- 1 teaspoon onion powder
- 2 garlic cloves, peeled and minced
- 2 lb. free range organic boneless skinless chicken breasts
- 2 tablespoons feta cheese
- 2 tablespoons ghee or olive oil
- Crushed red pepper to taste
- Salt and black pepper to taste

Directions:

- Preheat oven to 400oF. Place a cast-iron pan on medium high fire and heat for 5 minutes. Add oil and heat for 2 minutes more.
- Meanwhile in a large dish, mix well pepper, salt, crushed red pepper, paprika, coriander, and onion powder. Add chicken and coat well in seasoning.
- Add chicken to pan and brown sides for 4 minutes per side. Increase fire to high. Stir in garlic and onions. Lower fire to medium and mix well. Pop pan in oven and bake for 15 minutes.
- Remove from oven, turnover chicken and let it stand for 5 minutes before serving.

Nutritional Values: Calories 232; Carbs 5g; Fat 8g; Protein 33g

Spicy Chicken Leg Quarters

Serving Size: 3

Cooking Time: 53 minutes

Ingredients:

- 3 10-11 ozs. grass-fed bone-in, skin-on chicken leg quarters
- ½ cup mayonnaise
- 1 teaspoon paprika
- ½ teaspoon garlic powder
- Salt and ground white pepper, as required

Directions:

- Preheat the oven to 350 degrees. Generously, grease a baking dish.
- Add the mayonnaise in a shallow bowl.
- Place the paprika, garlic powder, salt and white pepper in a small bowl and mix well.
- Coat each chicken quarter with mayonnaise and then, sprinkle evenly with the spice mixture.
- Arrange the chicken quarters onto prepared baking sheet in a single layer.
- Bake for about 45 minutes.
- Now, increase the temperature of oven to 400 degrees F and bake for about 5-8 more minutes.
- Remove from oven and place the chicken quarters onto a platter.
- With a piece of foil, cover each chicken quarter loosely for about 5-10 minutes before serving.
- Serve.

Nutritional Values: Calories 325; Carbs 59.7g; Fat 1g; Protein 8.4g

Trout and Endives

Serving Size: 2

Cooking Time: 15 minutes

Ingredients:

- 4 trout fillets
- 2 endives, shredded
- ½ cup shallots, chopped
- 2 tablespoons olive oil
- 1 teaspoon rosemary, dried
- ¼ cup chicken stock
- A pinch of salt and black pepper
- 2 tablespoons chives, chopped

Directions:

- Heat up a large-sized pan with the oil over medium heat, add the shallots and the endives, toss and cook for 2 minutes.
- Add the fish and cook it for 2 minutes on each side.
- Add the rest of the prepared ingredients, cook for 8-9 minutes more, divide between plates and serve.

Nutritional Values: Calories 200; Carbs 2g; Fat 5g; Protein 7g

Chapter 3.
Dinner

Chicken and Mushrooms

Serving Size: 4

Cooking Time: 30 minutes

Ingredients:

- 1 pound chicken breast, skinless, boneless and cubed
- 2 cups baby bella mushrooms, sliced
- 2 tablespoons olive oil
- 1 red onion, chopped
- 1 red bell pepper, chopped
- 2 garlic cloves, minced
- A pinch of salt and black pepper
- ½ cup chicken stock
- 1 tablespoon balsamic vinegar
- 1 tablespoon parsley, chopped

Directions:

- Heat up a large-sized pan with the oil over medium heat, add the onion and the mushrooms, stir and cook for 5 minutes.
- Add the chicken, toss and brown for 5 minutes more.
- Add the rest of the prepared ingredients, toss, bring to a simmer and cook over medium heat for 20 minutes.
- Divide everything between plates and serve.

Nutritional Values: Calories 340; Carbs 4g; Fat 33g; Protein 20g

Hot Turkey Meatballs

Serving Size: 4

Cooking Time: 10 minutes

Ingredients:

- 1 pound turkey meat, ground
- 1 yellow onion, chopped
- 1 egg, whisked
- 1 tablespoon cilantro, chopped
- 1 tablespoon olive oil
- 1 red chili pepper, minced
- 1 teaspoon lime juice
- zest of 1 lime, grated
- a pinch of salt and black pepper
- 1 teaspoon turmeric powder

Directions:

- In a bowl, combine the turkey meat with the onion and the other ingredients except for the oil, stir & shape medium meatballs out of this mix.
- Heat up a pan with the oil over medium-high heat, add the meatballs, cook them for 5 minutes on each side, divide between plates, and serve for dinner.

Nutritional Values: Calories 200; Carbs 12g; Fat 12g; Protein 7g

Pasta with Alfredo Sauce

Serving Size: 2

Cooking Time: 25 minutes

Ingredients:

- Nonfat cooking spray
- 2 cloves of garlic, minced
- 2 tablespoons of fat-free cream cheese
- 1 1/3 cups of skim milk
- 2 tablespoons of all-purpose flour
- 2 tablespoons of butter sprinkles (or butter substitute)
- 1 cup of fat-free or low-fat Parmesan cheese
- Black pepper, to taste
- 2 cups of cooked pasta of choice

Directions:

- Spray nonstick skillet with cooking spray. Add garlic over low heat and cook until tender.
- Add cream cheese, milk, and flour, whisking over medium heat; bring to a boil.
- Reduce heat to an actual simmer and cook until sauce has thickened.
- Add butter sprinkles, Parmesan cheese, and black pepper, whisk until combined. Immediately add to pasta and toss to coat.

Nutritional Values: Calories 440; Carbs 60g; Fat 1.5g; Protein 27g

Seared Haddocks with Beets

Serving Size: 4

Cooking Time: 30 minutes

Ingredients:

- 8 beets, peeled and cut into eighths
- 2 shallots, thinly sliced
- 2 tablespoons apple cider vinegar
- 2 tablespoons olive oil, divided
- 1 teaspoon bottled minced garlic
- 1 teaspoon chopped fresh thyme
- Pinch sea salt
- 4 (5-ounce / 142-g) haddock fillets, patted dry

Directions:

- Preheat the oven to a heat of 400°F (205°C).
- Combine the beets, shallots, vinegar, 1 tablespoon of olive oil, garlic, thyme, and sea salt in a medium bowl, and toss to coat well. Spread out the beet mixture in a baking dish.
- Roast in the preheated oven for approximately about 30 minutes, turning once or twice with a spatula, or until the beets are tender.
- Meanwhile, heat the remaining 1 tablespoon of the prepared olive oil in a large skillet over medium-high heat.
- Add the haddock and sear each side for 4 to 5 minutes, or until the flesh is opaque and it flakes apart easily.
- Transfer the fish to a plate and serve topped with the roasted beets.

Nutritional Values: Calories 343; Fat 8.8g; Carbohydrates 20.9g; Protein 38.1g

Turkey Artichokes

Serving Size: 4

Cooking Time: 40 minutes

Ingredients:

- 1 yellow onion, sliced
- 1 pound turkey breast, skinless, boneless, and roughly cubed
- 1 tablespoon olive oil
- salt and black pepper to taste
- 1 cup of canned artichoke hearts, drained and halved
- ½ teaspoon nutmeg, ground
- ½ teaspoon sweet paprika
- 1 teaspoon cumin, ground
- 1 tablespoon cilantro, chopped

Directions:

- In a roasting pan, combine the turkey with the onion, artichokes, and the other ingredients, toss and at 350°F for 40 minutes.
- Divide everything between plates and serve.

Nutritional Values: Calories 345; Fat 12g; Carbohydrates 12g; Protein 14g

Chapter 4.
Snacks

Fiery Shrimp Cocktail Salad

Serving Size: 4

Cooking Time: 15 minutes

Ingredients:

- 2 tablespoon olive oil 1/2 head Romaine lettuce, torn
- 1 cucumber, cut into ribbons
- 1/2 lb shrimp, deveined
- 1 cup of arugula
- 1/2 cup mayonnaise
- 2 tablespoon Cholula hot sauce
- 1/2 teaspoon Worcestershire sauce
- Chili pepper and salt to taste
- 1 2 tablespoon lemon juice
- 1 lemon Cut into wedges
- 4 Dill Weed

Directions:

- Sprinkle the shrimp with salt and pepper. Heat the prepared olive oil on moderate heat, and fry for three minutes per side until opaque and pink. Place the shrimp aside to cool.
- Mix your mayonnaise mix, juice of a hot lemon sauce, and Worcestershire sauce in a bowl, mixing until it is smooth and creamy in the bowl. Divide the cucumber and lettuce into four glass bowls. Serve with shrimp, then pour the hot dressing on top. Sprinkle arugula all over and garnish using lemon wedges and dill. Serve.

Nutritional Values: Calories 241; Carbs 3.9g; Fat 18g; Protein 14g

Honey Granola

Serving Size: 8

Cooking Time: 30 minutes

Ingredients:

- 4 cups oatmeal
- 1 cup flaked or shredded unsweetened coconut
- 1 cup raw, hulled sunflower seeds
- 1 cup chopped walnuts
- ½ cup raw wheat germ
- ¼ cup flaxseed meal
- ¼ cup oil (canola or olive)
- ¼ cup pasteurized honey

Directions:

- Preheat oven to 350°F.
- In a large bowl, mix oatmeal, coconut, sunflower seeds, walnuts, wheat germ, and flaxseed meal.
- Combine oil and honey in microwaveable container and add a splash of water. Microwave for 15 seconds, then stir to combine thoroughly.
- Pour honey mixture over dry ingredients in bowl, stir thoroughly to coat granola.
- Spread mixture evenly on 2 cookie sheets and bake for 30 minutes or until granola reaches desired crunchiness. Use a spatula to stir granola every few minutes.
- Allow to actually cool on cookie sheet, then store in an airtight container.

Nutritional Values: Calories 150; Carbs 15g; Fat 9g; Protein 4g

Pesto Veggie Pinwheels

Serving Size: 4

Cooking Time: 40 minutes

Ingredients:

- 3 whole eggs
- 1 egg, beaten for brushing
- 1 cup grated cheese
- 1 cup of almond flour
- 3 tablespoons coconut flour
- 1/2 teaspoon 1 teaspoon
- 4 tablespoon cream cheese, softened
- 1/4 teaspoon yogurt
- One cup of cold butter
- 1 cup of mushrooms, chopped
- 1 cup basil pesto
- 2 cups baby spinach
- Salt to taste

Directions:

- Mix coconut and almond flour, Xanthan gum, and 1/2 teaspoon salt in a bowl. Add cream cheese, yogurt, and butter; mix until it is crumbly. Incorporate three eggs in succession and mix until the dough is formed into an oval. Make the dough flat on a flat, clean surface, wrap it in plastic wrap and chill for an hour.

- Dust a clean, flat area with almond flour. Cut off the dough and then roll out to 15x12 inches. Spread pesto over the top using a spatula, leaving a 2-inch border along one side. A bowl mixes baby mushrooms and spinach, season with salt and black pepper, and spreads the mixture on top of the pesto. Sprinkle with cheese, and wrap as tightly as possible, starting at the lower end. Refrigerate for 10 minutes. Preheat the oven to 350 F. Take the pastry from the fridge onto a flat surface, and then use the sharp edge of a knife, cut it into 24 small discs. Lay them out in a baking tray, brush with the remaining egg and bake for about 25 minutes until they are golden. Allow cooling.

Nutritional Values: Calories 241; Carbs 3.4g; Fat 39g; Protein 20g

Spinach Chips with Avocado Hummus

Serving Size: 4

Cooking Time: 25 minutes

Ingredients:

- 1 tbsp olive oil
- 1/2 cup baby spinach
- 1/2 tsp plain vinegar
- 3 avocados, chopped
- Half cup chopped parsley
- 1/2 cup butter
- 1 cup of pumpkin seeds
- 1/4 cup sesame paste
- Juice from half a lemon
- 1 clove of garlic, minced
- 1/2 teaspoon coriander powder
- Black pepper and salt to taste

Directions:

- Preheat the oven to 350 F. Place leaves in bowls and mix in simple vinegar, olive oil, and salt. Spread the spinach on a parchment-lined baking tray and bake till the leaves are crisp but not burnt, about 15 minutes.
- Place the avocados into the food processor. Add pumpkin seeds, butter, sesame paste, garlic, lemon juice, coriander, salt, and pepper. Puree until smooth. Serve in a large-sized bowl and garnish with chopped parsley. Serve with chips of spinach.

Nutritional Values: Calories 348; Carbs 7g; Fat 5g; Protein 10g

Sweet Butternut

Serving Size: 8

Cooking Time: 4 hours

Ingredients:

- 1 cup carrots, chopped
- 1 tablespoon olive oil
- 1 yellow onion, chopped
- 1/2 teaspoon stevia
- 1 garlic clove, minced
- 1/2 teaspoon curry powder
- 1 butternut squash, cubed
- 2 and 1/2 cups low-sodium veggie stock
- 1/2 cup basmati rice
- ¾ cup coconut milk
- 1/2 teaspoon cinnamon powder
- 1/4 teaspoon ginger, grated

Directions:

- Heat up a pan with the oil over medium-high heat, add the oil, onion, garlic, stevia, carrots, curry powder, cinnamon and ginger, stir, cook for 5 minutes and transfer to your slow cooker.
- Add squash, stock and coconut milk, stir, cover and cook on Low for 4 hours.
- Divide the butternut mix between plates and serve as a side dish.

Nutritional Values: Calories 134; Carbs 16.5g; Fat 7.2g; Protein 1.8g

Chapter 5.
Soups and Side Dishes

Butternut Squash Soup

Serving Size: 8

Cooking Time: 40 minutes

Ingredients:

- 2 tablespoons of olive oil
- ⅔ cup of onions, finely chopped
- 1 cup of carrots, thinly sliced
- 1 large potato, peeled, cubed
- 2 cups of butternut squash, peeled, cubed
- 1 Granny Smith apple, peeled, cored, cubed
- 4 cups of chicken broth
- ¼ teaspoon of nutmeg
- salt and pepper to taste
- ½ cup of milk (optional)

Directions:

- Warm the prepared olive oil in a medium saucepan, then add the onions and continue to cook them over low heat for approximately 5 minutes, or until they have softened.
- After adding the carrots, potato, squash, apple, and chicken broth, simmer everything covered over a low heat for approximately about half an hour, or until the veggies are soft. Stir in nutmeg, salt and pepper.
- Put one-half of the ingredients in a blender and process until completely smooth. Transfer the contents of the first saucepan or big bowl to a second saucepan or bowl, and then combine the second half of the veggies until smooth.
- Place back into the pot and, if desired, whisk with some milk. Serve.

Nutritional Values: Calories 100; Carbs 29g; Fat 2.5g; Protein 2g

Classic Tabbouleh

Serving Size: 4

Cooking Time: 10 minutes

Ingredients:

- ¾ cup bulgur
- 2 cups freshly chopped parsley
- 1½ cups water
- ½ cup fresh lemon juice
- ½ cup extra-virgin olive oil
- ½ red bell pepper, diced
- 3 ripe plum tomatoes, peeled, seeded, and diced
- 1 large cucumber, peeled, seeded, and diced
- ¾ cup chopped scallions, white and green parts
- ½ green bell pepper, diced
- ½ cup finely chopped fresh mint
- A handful of greens for serving
- Seasoned pita wedges
- Sea salt to taste
- Freshly ground pepper to taste

Directions:

- Preheat the oven to around 375°F.
- Take a medium-sized bowl and add the asparagus with 2 tablespoons of salt and olive oil.
- Take out a baking dish and add the asparagus. Place the tray in the oven, then roast for about 10 minutes, or until the asparagus becomes tender.
- Take out the asparagus and set it aside.
- Use another medium-sized bowl and add garlic, lime juice, orange juice, and the remaining 2 tablespoons of olive oil. Whisk all the ingredients together. Add salt and pepper to taste.
- Take the lettuce and split it into 6 plates. Take out the asparagus and place it on top of the lettuce.
- Pour the dressing over the asparagus and lettuce salad. Top the salad with basil and pine nuts. Add a small amount of Romano cheese for garnish, if you prefer.
- In the oven, you can toast the pine nuts as well. Use the method below:
- Prepare a baking pan with a nonstick baking sheet. Add the pine nuts on top.
- Bake at 375°F for about 5-10 minutes, or until the nuts are lightly browned.
- Take from the oven, then set aside to cool.
- Add the nuts to the salad as a topping.

Nutritional Values: Calories 177; Carbs 28g; Fat 11g; Protein 12g

Crispy Herb Cauliflower Florets

Serving Size: 2

Cooking Time: 20 minutes

Ingredients:

- 1 egg, beaten
- 2 tablespoons parmesan cheese, grated
- 2 cups cauliflower florets, boiled
- ¼ cup almond flour
- 1 tablespoon olive oil
- Salt to taste
- ½ tablespoon mixed herbs
- ½ teaspoon chili powder
- ½ teaspoon garlic powder
- ½ cup breadcrumbs

Directions:

- Combine garlic powder, breadcrumbs, chili powder, mixed herbs, salt, and cheese in a bowl.
- Stir the olive oil into the breadcrumb mixture well.
- Place flour in a bowl and place the egg in another bowl.
- Dip the cauliflower florets into the beaten egg, then in flour, and coat with breadcrumbs.
- Preheat your air fryer to 350°Fahrenheit.
- Place the coated cauliflower florets inside the air fryer basket and cook for 20-minutes.

Nutritional Values: Calories 253; Carbs 9.5g; Fat 11.3g; Protein 8.5g

White Bean Soup

Serving Size: 6

Cooking Time: 8 hours

Ingredients:

- 1 cup celery, chopped
- 1 cup carrots, chopped
- 1 yellow onion, chopped
- 6 cups veggie stock
- 4 garlic cloves, minced
- 2 cup navy beans, dried
- ½ teaspoon basil, dried
- ½ teaspoon sage, dried
- 1 teaspoon thyme, dried
- A pinch of salt and black pepper

Directions:

- In your slow cooker, combine the beans with the stock and the rest of the ingredients, put the lid on, and cook on Low for 8 hours.
- Divide the soup into bowls and serve right away.

Nutritional Values: Calories 264; Carbs 23.7g; Fat 17.5g; Protein 11.5g

Wonton Soup

Serving Size: 8

Cooking Time: 25 minutes

Ingredients:

- 1 recipe of Asian Broth
- 2½ cups Napa cabbage leaves, core removed and chopped
- 1 pound lean ground pork
- 1/3 cup green onions, chopped
- ¼ teaspoon garlic powder
- ¼ teaspoon onion powder
- ½ teaspoon low-sodium soy sauce
- ½ cup water chestnuts, chopped
- 1 package wonton wrappers
- 3 tablespoons egg substitute

Directions:

- Preheat oven to 400°F.
- Place broth and cabbage in a deep pan and bring to a simmer.
- Combine pork, green onions, garlic powder, onion powder, soy sauce, egg substitute, water chestnuts, and 2 cups of cooked cabbage.
- Mix well to combine and form into teaspoon-size balls.
- Place balls on parchment-lined sheet pan and bake in oven for 5 minutes. Remove from oven and allow to cool.
- Once cooled, place meatball in wonton wrapper; fold into a triangle and seal edges of the wrappers by moistening with water and pressing the edges together firmly.
- Place in simmering broth and cook 3 to 4 minutes until they float. Serve immediately.

Nutritional Values: Calories 320; Carbs 34g; Fat 13g; Protein 16g

30-Day Meal Plan

Day	Breakfast	Lunch	Dinner
1	Turkey Caprese Meatloaf Cups	Paprika and Feta Cheese on Chicken Skillet	Seared Haddocks with Beets
2	Apple Pancakes	Balsamic Chicken and Beans	Pasta with Alfredo Sauce
3	Roasted Root Vegetable Hash	Spicy Chicken Leg Quarters	Hot Turkey Meatballs
4	Baked Beans	Paprika and Feta Cheese on Chicken Skillet	Seared Haddocks with Beets
5	Veggie Omelet	Balsamic Chicken and Beans	Hot Turkey Meatballs
6	Turkey Caprese Meatloaf Cups	Spicy Chicken Leg Quarters	Turkey Artichokes
7	Baked Beans	Trout and Endives	Pasta with Alfredo Sauce
8	Roasted Root Vegetable Hash	Lavender Lamb Chops	Chicken and Mushrooms
9	Veggie Omelet	Trout and Endives	Hot Turkey Meatballs
10	Apple Pancakes	Spicy Chicken Leg Quarters	Turkey Artichokes
11	Veggie Omelet	Lavender Lamb Chops	Chicken and Mushrooms
12	Roasted Root Vegetable Hash	Balsamic Chicken and Beans	Turkey Artichokes
13	Baked Beans	Paprika and Feta Cheese on Chicken Skillet	Pasta with Alfredo Sauce
14	Turkey Caprese Meatloaf Cups	Spicy Chicken Leg Quarters	Hot Turkey Meatballs
15	Apple Pancakes	Paprika and Feta Cheese on Chicken Skillet	Seared Haddocks with Beets

16	Baked Beans	Trout and Endives	Pasta with Alfredo Sauce
17	Veggie Omelet	Balsamic Chicken and Beans	Turkey Artichokes
18	Roasted Root Vegetable Hash	Spicy Chicken Leg Quarters	Chicken and Mushrooms
19	Apple Pancakes	Lavender Lamb Chops	Seared Haddocks with Beets
20	Veggie Omelet	Paprika and Feta Cheese on Chicken Skillet	Turkey Artichokes
21	Turkey Caprese Meatloaf Cups	Trout and Endives	Hot Turkey Meatballs
22	Veggie Omelet	Lavender Lamb Chops	Turkey Artichokes
23	Apple Pancakes	Trout and Endives	Pasta with Alfredo Sauce
24	Roasted Root Vegetable Hash	Spicy Chicken Leg Quarters	Chicken and Mushrooms
25	Baked Beans	Lavender Lamb Chops	Seared Haddocks with Beets
26	Turkey Caprese Meatloaf Cups	Balsamic Chicken and Beans	Pasta with Alfredo Sauce
27	Roasted Root Vegetable Hash	Paprika and Feta Cheese on Chicken Skillet	Hot Turkey Meatballs
28	Turkey Caprese Meatloaf Cups	Spicy Chicken Leg Quarters	Chicken and Mushrooms
29	Apple Pancakes	Balsamic Chicken and Beans	Seared Haddocks with Beets
30	Baked Beans	Lavender Lamb Chops	Chicken and Mushrooms

BOOK 4.
DR. NOWZARADAN'S MEAL PLAN ON A BUDGET

Introduction

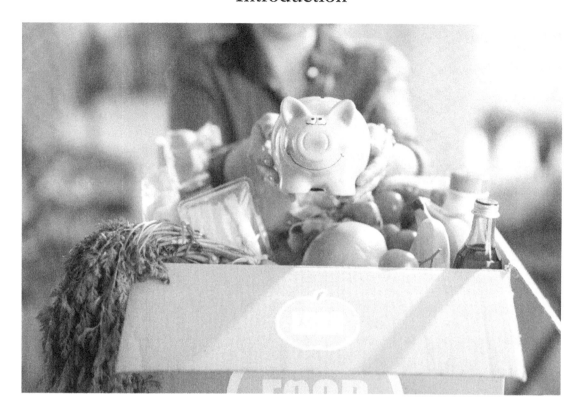

The Dr. Nowzaradan diet, or Dr. Now diet, is a 1,000-1,200 calorie diet designed to promote rapid weight, it is suitable for every weight and stage of life. This 1,200 calorie diet plan contains too many moments to demonstrate and detail on a weight loss program that helps you lose up to 20 pounds, pounds on your self, and it means you live a happier and more proft life.

This diet has been customized for those of you who are not in good health, although it can also be implemented for people who want to recover their well-being and for those who want to lose weight. It consists of 1200 calories and includes a number of recipes. These recipes are easy-to-find ingredients and ensure that you're getting the vitamins you need from food. It also includes an exercise plan in free-lance.

This book will show you how to eliminate the harmful elements in your life and replace them with healthier options. My diet plan is uniquely designed to help you reach your ideal weight (provided you follow the plan). This plan will help you lose 1 to 2 pounds a week until you reach your ideal weight. This is a lifestyle you can manage; it will allow you to eat healthy foods while meeting your caloric needs. And it will help to keep you from becoming hungry and stressed out. A better alternative to weight loss is to gradually develop healthy lifestyle behaviors that you can maintain long-term, such as increasing your intake of fruits and vegetables, prioritizing sleep, and staying physically active.

Chapter 1.
Breakfast

Brussels Sprouts Delight

Serving Size: 3

Cooking Time: 12 minutes

Ingredients:

- 3 eggs
- Salt and black pepper to the taste
- 1 tablespoon ghee, melted
- 2 shallots, minced
- 2 garlic cloves, minced
- 12 ounces Brussels sprouts, thinly sliced
- 2 ounces bacon, chopped
- 1 and ½ tablespoons apple cider vinegar

Directions:

- Heat up a large-sized pan over medium heat, add bacon, stir, cook until it's crispy, transfer to a plate and leave aside for now.
- Heat up the large-sized pan again over medium heat, add shallots and garlic, stir and cook for 30 seconds.
- Add Brussels sprouts, salt, pepper and apple cider vinegar, stir and cook for 5 minutes.
- Return bacon to pan, stir and cook for 5 minutes more.
- Add ghee, stir and make a hole in the center.
- Crack eggs into the pan, cook until they are done and serve right away.
- Enjoy!

Nutritional Values: Calories 240; Fat 7g; Carbohydrates 7g; Protein 12g

Cauliflower Based Waffles

Serving Size: 2

Cooking Time: 25 minutes

Ingredients:

- 1 cup zucchini chopped and squeezed
- 2 green onions
- 1 tablespoon olive oil
- 2 eggs
- 1/3 cup Parmesan cheese
- 1 cup mozzarella, grated
- Half head cauliflower
- 1 teaspoon garlic powder
- 1 tablespoon sesame seeds
- 2 teaspoons thyme, chopped

Directions:

- Cut the cauliflower into florets. Mix the pieces in the food processor and then pulse until rice is created. Return to your food processor, and add the zucchini, green onions and thyme. Pulse until smooth.
- Transfer into an empty bowl. Add all the other prepared ingredients and mix well. Allow sitting for 10 mins. Warm the waffle iron, then spread it all over the mixture. Cook until golden brown in about 5 minutes.

Nutritional Values: Calories 316; Carbs 7.2g; Fat 21g; Protein 32g

Eggs and Veggies

Serving Size: 4

Cooking Time: 10 minutes

Ingredients:

- 2 tomatoes, chopped
- 2 eggs, beaten
- 1 bell pepper, chopped
- 1 teaspoon tomato paste
- ¼ cup of water
- 1 teaspoon butter
- ½ white onion, diced
- ½ teaspoon chili flakes
- 1/3 teaspoon sea salt

Directions:

- Put butter in the large-sized pan and melt it. Add bell pepper and cook it for approximately about 3 minutes over the medium heat. Stir it from time to time.
- After this, add the prepared diced onion and cook it for approximately about 2 minutes more. Stir the vegetables and add tomatoes.
- Cook them for 5 minutes over the medium-low heat. Then add water and tomato paste. Stir well. Add prepared beaten eggs, chili flakes, and sea salt.
- Stir well and cook menemen for 4 minutes over the medium-low heat.
- The cooked meal should be half runny.

Nutritional Values: Calories 67; Carbs 6.4g; Fat 3.4g; Protein 3.8g

Spiced Oatmeal

Serving Size: 4

Cooking Time: 9 hours

Ingredients:

- 1 cup steel cut oats
- 2 tablespoons stevia
- ½ teaspoon cinnamon powder
- A pinch of cloves, ground
- ½ cup pumpkin puree
- 4 cups water
- Olive oil cooking spray
- ½ cup fat-free milk
- A pinch of nutmeg, ground
- A pinch of allspice, ground
- A pinch of ginger, ground

Directions:

- Grease your slow cooker with the cooking spray, add the oats, the pumpkin puree, water, milk, stevia, cinnamon, cloves, allspice, ginger and nutmeg, cover and cook on Low for 9 hours.
- Stir the oatmeal, divide it into bowls and serve.

Nutritional Values: Calories 200; Carbs 25.5g; Fat 1.5g; Protein 4g

Zucchini Skilletcakes

Serving Size: 8

Cooking Time: 8 minutes

Ingredients:

- 12 tablespoons. alkaline water
- 6 large grated zucchinis
- Sea salt
- 4 tablespoons. ground Flax Seeds
- 2 teaspoons. olive oil
- 2 finely chopped jalapeño peppers
- 1/2 cup finely chopped scallions

Directions:

- In a container, mix together water and the flax seeds then set it aside.
- Pour oil in a large non-stick skillet then heat it on medium heat.
- The add the black pepper, salt, and zucchini.
- Cook for 3 minutes then transfer the zucchini into a large container.
- Add the flax seed and the scallion's mixture then properly mix it.
- Preheat a griddle then grease it lightly with the cooking spray.
- Pour 1/4 of the zucchini mixture into griddle then cook for 3 minutes.
- Flip the side carefully then cook for 2 more minutes.
- Repeat the procedure with the remaining mixture in batches.
- Serve.

Nutritional Values: Calories 271; Carbs 9.8g; Fat 2.8g; Protein 3g

Chapter 2.
Lunch

Cashew Chicken Curry

Serving Size: 4

Cooking Time: 25 minutes

Ingredients:

- 1 cups Cauliflower
- 2 large fresh tomatoes
- 1 medium red onion
- 2 cups Cucumber
- 2 tablespoon Coconut oil
- 1 lb. Breasts of chicken
- 1 large Egg white
- For the Garnish:
- Freshly chopped fresh mint
- Minced fresh cilantro
- Food processor & Rimmed baking sheet

Directions:

- Chop the cauliflower into florets and quarter the tomatoes. Roughly chop the onion and thinly slice the cucumber into halves. Take off the skin and bones from the chicken.
- Heat the oven to 425° Fahrenheit.
- Toss the quartered tomatoes, cauliflower florets, and onion into a mixing container. Melt the coconut oil and sprinkle using 1.5 teaspoons of curry powder. Mix until well.
- Prepare on a baking sheet in one layer. Dust with pepper and salt to your liking. Add the rest of the curry powder and cashews into a food processor. Pulse leaving a few chunks for texture.
- Pat to remove the moisture from the chicken breasts using a paper towel.
- Put the egg white and cashews into two shallow plates.
- Dredge the chicken through the egg white. Shake off any excess and press into the cashews.
- Flip and lightly press the other side into the cashews.
- Put the chicken breast onto a small cooling rack that fits on your sheet pan (one with legs is preferred, so it sits over the veggies).
- Continue the process with the remaining chicken. Place the cooling rack over a sheet pan (over the top of the veggies).
- Bake the chicken to reach an internal temperature of 165° Fahrenheit (14-15 min.). Once it's done, toss the fresh cucumbers onto the pan.

Garnish with mint and cilantro.

Nutritional Values: Calories 364; Fat 18g; Carbohydrates 14g; Protein 34g

Honey Balsamic Salmon and Lemon Asparagus

Serving Size: 4

Cooking Time: 10 minutes

Ingredients:

- 2 tablespoon balsamic vinegar
- 1 tablespoon raw honey
- 1 teaspoon sea salt, divided
- 1/2 teaspoon freshly ground black pepper
- 4 salmon filets (about 2 1/2 lb total)
- 1 1/2 cups water, divided
- 1 bunch asparagus, trimmed and halved
- 2 tablespoon ghee
- Juice of 1 lemon

Directions:

- In a bowl, whisk the vinegar, honey, 1/2 teaspoon salt, and the pepper to combine. Drizzle the honey-vinegar mixture over the salmon, and using the back of the spoon, spread it evenly across the salmon. Place a metal trivet or steam rack in the Instant Pot and pour in 1 cup of water. Place the salmon on the trivet, skin-side down. Lock the lid.
- Select Pressure Cook mode and cook at high pressure for 3 minutes.
- When cooking is complete, use a quick release. Remove the lid. Using potholders, remove the trivet and salmon filets, transfer the fish to a serving platter or glass dish, and cover with aluminum foil. Set aside. Select Cancel. Put the asparagus, the remaining 1/2 cup of water, the ghee, and the remaining 1/2 teaspoon salt into the Instant Pot. Lock the lid.
- Select Pressure Cook mode and cook at high pressure for 2 minutes. When cooking is complete, use a quick release. Remove the lid and transfer the cooked asparagus to the serving platter with the fish. Pour the lemon juice over the asparagus and fish and serve.

Nutritional Values: Calories 444; Carbs 11g; Fat 18g; Protein 57g

Miso Chicken with Sesame

Serving Size: 6

Cooking Time: 4 hours

Ingredients:

- ¼ cup white miso
- 2 tablespoons coconut oil, melted
- 2 tablespoons honey
- 1 tablespoon rice wine vinegar, unseasoned
- 2 garlic cloves, thinly sliced
- 1 teaspoon fresh ginger root, minced
- 1 cup chicken broth
- 8 boneless, skinless chicken thighs
- 2 scallions, sliced
- 1 tablespoon sesame seeds

Directions:

- Combine the miso, coconut oil, honey, rice wine vinegar, garlic, and ginger root in a slow cooker. Mix it well.
- Add the chicken and toss to combine. Cover and cook on high for approximately about 4 hours.
- Transfer the chicken and sauce to a serving dish. Garnish with the scallions and sesame seeds and serve.

Nutritional Values: Calories 320; Carbs 17g; Fat 15g; Protein 32g

Spaghetti Bolognese

Serving Size: 8

Cooking Time: 20 minutes

Ingredients:

- 1 lb brown rice spaghetti
- 2 tablespoon ghee
- 3 garlic cloves, minced
- 1/2 cup chopped white onion
- 2/3 cup chopped celery
- 2/3 cup chopped carrot
- 1 lb lean ground beef
- 1 (15-oz) can of diced tomatoes with their juice
- 1 tablespoon white wine vinegar
- 1/2 teaspoon red pepper flakes
- 1/8 teaspoon ground nutmeg
- Dash salt
- Dash freshly ground black pepper

Directions:

- Cook the spaghetti following the package instructions.
- Meanwhile, in a large-sized skillet over medium heat, heat the ghee.
- Add the prepared garlic and onion, and sauté for 5 minutes. Add the celery and carrot, and sauté for 5 minutes. Push the vegetables to the side of the skillet.
- Add the ground beef next to the vegetables. Sauté for 10 minutes, breaking up the meat as it begins to brown. Stir in the tomatoes, vinegar, red pepper flakes, nutmeg, salt, and pepper, and bring to a simmer for 5 minutes. Serve over the cooked noodles.

Nutritional Values: Calories 358; Carbs 48g; Fat 12g; Protein 14g

Veal Parmesan

Serving Size: 6

Cooking Time: 1 hour 10 minutes

Ingredients:

- 8 veal cutlets
- 2/3 cup parmesan, grated
- 8 provolone cheese slices
- Salt and black pepper to the taste
- 5 cups tomato sauce
- A pinch of garlic salt
- Cooking spray
- 2 tablespoons ghee
- 2 tablespoons coconut oil, melted
- 1 teaspoon Italian seasoning

Directions:

- Season veal cutlets with salt, pepper and garlic salt an drub,
- Heat up a pan with the ghee and the oil over medium high heat, add veal and cook until they brown on all sides.
- Spread half of the tomato sauce on the bottom of a baking dish which you've greased with some cooking spray.
- Add veal cutlets, then sprinkle Italian seasoning and spread the rest of the sauce.
- Cover dish, introduce in the oven at 350 degrees F and bake for 40 minutes.
- Uncover dish, spread provolone cheese and sprinkle parmesan, introduce in the oven again and bake for 15 minutes more.
- Divide on plates and serve. Enjoy!

Nutritional Values: Calories 362; Carbs 6g; Fat 21g; Protein 26g

Chapter 2.
Dinner

Bell Peppers and Sausage

Serving Size: 4

Cooking Time: 10 minutes

Ingredients:

- ¾-cup tomato spaghetti sauce
- 5-oz. mozzarella cheese, grated.
- 1 large red pepper, thickly sliced.
- 6-oz. onion, chopped.
- 1¼-lbs. Italian sausages.
- 2-tablespoon olive oil
- 1 large green bell pepper, chunked.
- 2 cloves garlic, finely chopped

Directions:

- Brown the sausages in a skillet over a medium heat. When the sausages are partially cooked add in the peppers, onion and garlic
- Continue to actually cook until the sausages are done and the vegetables are still crisp. Take the sausages out of the skillet and slice into chunky bite sized pieces. Return to the pan
- Stir in the spaghetti sauce and cover. Simmer for approximately about 5 to 8 minutes until all is piping hot. Sprinkle with the cheese and serve.

Nutritional Values: Calories 434; Carbs 18g; Fat 60g; Protein 21.6g

Brown Rice Pilaf with Butternut Squash

Serving Size: 3

Cooking Time: 50 minutes

Ingredients:

- Pepper to taste
- A pinch of cinnamon
- 1 teaspoon salt
- 2 tablespoon chopped fresh oregano
- ½ cup chopped fennel fronds
- ½ cup white wine
- 1 ¾ cups water + 2 tablespoon, divided
- 1 cup instant or parboiled brown rice
- 1 tablespoon tomato paste
- 1 garlic clove, minced
- 1 large onion, finely chopped
- 3 tablespoon extra virgin olive oil
- 2 lbs. butternut squash, halved

Directions:

- In a large hole grater, grate squash.
- On medium low fire, place a large nonstick skillet and heat oil for 2 minutes.
- Add garlic and onions. Sauté for 8 minutes or until lightly colored and soft.
- Add 2 tablespoon water and tomato paste. Stir well to combine and cook for approximately about 3 minutes. Add rice, mix well to coat in mixture and cook for 5 minutes while stirring frequently. If needed, add squash in batches until it has wilted so that you can cover pan.
- Add remaining water and increase fire to medium high. Add wine, cover and boil. Once boiling, lower fire to an actual simmer and cook for 20 to 25 minutes or until liquid is fully absorbed. Stir in pepper, cinnamon, salt, oregano, and fennel fronds.
- Turn off fire, cover and let it stand for 5 minutes before serving.

Nutritional Values: Calories 147; Carbs 22.1g; Fat 5.5g; Protein 2.3g

Green Bean Casserole

Serving Size: 8

Cooking Time: 25 minutes

Ingredients:

- ½ yellow onion, sliced thin
- 2 tablespoons of butter
- 1 cup of bread crumbs
- ½ cup of low-fat Parmesan cheese
- 1 cup of low-fat or fat-free cream of mushroom soup
- ½ cup of skim milk
- 1 teaspoon of soy sauce
- Fresh ground black pepper
- 4 cups of cut green beans, frozen and thawed
- 1 tablespoon of dry thyme

Directions:

- Sauté onions in butter and add bread crumbs and Parmesan.
- Mix all remaining ingredients together and pour into a casserole dish.
- Cover with bread crumbs and onion mixture and bake for 20–25 minutes.

Nutritional Values: Calories 350; Carbs 20g; Fat 6g; Protein 6g

Nut-Crusted Chicken Breasts

Serving Size: 4

Cooking Time: 20 minutes

Ingredients:

- 2 boneless, skinless chicken breasts, lightly pounded to even thickness
- ¼ cup of flour
- 3 ounces of liquid egg replacement
- Salt and pepper, to taste
- ¼ teaspoon of cinnamon
- ¼ teaspoon of dry thyme
- ¼ teaspoon of dry mustard
- 1/8 teaspoon of cayenne
- ½ cup of very finely chopped pistachios, walnuts, almonds, or pecans
- 2 tablespoons of canola oil
- 4 tablespoons of maple syrup
- 1 tablespoon of Dijon mustard

Directions:

- Lightly dust chicken in flour and coat in beaten egg replacement. In a medium bowl, combine salt and pepper, cinnamon, thyme, dry mustard, and cayenne with the chopped nuts.
- Dredge (dip) chicken into nut mixture and press to completely cover the chicken.
- Place oil in nonstick pan and heat over medium heat.
- Place chicken in pan and cook until nuts brown (2–3 minutes), flip and cook for 2–3 minutes on second side, then place chicken in oven for 5–7 minutes.
- Pour over chicken for the last 2 minutes in the oven.

Nutritional Values: Calories 320; Carbs 20g; Fat 16g; Protein 20g

Tangy Chicken Drumsticks

Serving Size: 5

Cooking Time: 1 hour 15 minutes

Ingredients:

- 2 tablespoons olive oil
- 2 lbs. chicken drumsticks, boneless, skinless
- Sea salt and ground black pepper, to taste
- 2 garlic cloves, minced
- 1/2 cup tomato paste
- 1/2 cup chicken broth
- 4 tablespoons rice vinegar
- 2 scallions, chopped

Directions:

- Start by preheating the oven to 330 degrees F. Brush the sides and bottom of a baking pan with olive oil.
- Arrange the chicken drumsticks in the baking pan. Add the salt, black pepper, garlic, tomato paste, chicken broth, and rice vinegar to the pan.
- Bake for approximately about 1 hour 10 minutes or until everything is heated through.
- Garnish with scallions and serve. Bon appétit!

Nutritional Values: Calories 352; Carbs 2g; Fat 22.1g; Protein 33g

Chapter 3.
Snacks

Avocado Tuna Bites

Serving Size: 4

Cooking Time: 5 minutes

Ingredients:

- 1/3 cup coconut oil
- 1 avocado, cut into cubes
- 10 ounces canned tuna, drained
- ¼ cup parmesan cheese, grated
- ¼ teaspoon garlic powder
- 1/4 teaspoon onion powder
- 1/3 cup almond flour
- ¼ teaspoon pepper
- ¼ cup low fat mayonnaise
- Pepper as needed

Directions:

- Take a bowl and add tuna, mayo, flour, parmesan, spices and mix well.
- Fold in avocado and make 12 balls out of the mixture.
- Melt coconut oil in pan and cook over medium heat, until all sides are golden.
- Serve and enjoy!

Nutritional Values: Calories 205; Carbs 1g; Fat 18g; Protein 5g

Chicken Salad with Parmesan

Serving Size: 2

Cooking Time: 30 minutes

Ingredients:

- 1 lb breast of chicken chopped
- 1 cup juice of a lemon
- 2 cloves of garlic, minced
- 2 tablespoons olive oil
- 1 Romaine lettuce, chopped
- 3 Parmesan crisps
- 2 tablespoon Parmesan Grated Dressing
- 2 tablespoons extra olive oil
- 1 tablespoon lemon juice
- Black pepper and salt to taste

Directions:

- Add the chicken with lemon juice, oil, and garlic to the Ziploc bag. Close in the bag, shake it to blend, and chill for one hour. The grill should be heated to medium, and grill the chicken for approximately 3-4 minutes on each side.
- Mix the dressing ingredients in one bowl, and mix thoroughly on a serving plate layout, with salad leaves and Parmesan crisps. Sprinkle the dressing over them and then toss in a coating. Add Chicken and Parmesan cheese. Serve.

Nutritional Values: Calories 329; Carbs 5g; Fat 32g; Protein 34g

Creamed Peas

Serving Size: 4

Cooking Time: 25 minutes

Ingredients:

- ⅔ cup of chicken broth
- 2 cups of green peas
- 2 tablespoons of butter
- ⅓ cup of half-and-half
- 2 tablespoons of flour
- ¼ teaspoon of black pepper
- ¼ teaspoon of salt
- 2 tablespoons of Parmesan cheese, grated (optional)

Directions:

- In a medium saucepan, add broth and peas; bring to near boiling. Reduce heat.
- Cover; cook on low heat 25 minutes, or until peas are tender. Add butter.
- In a small-sized bowl, combine half-and-half and flour; add to the peas mixture, cook and stir until thickened.
- Add the pepper and salt, plus Parmesan cheese if desired, stirring to combine.

Nutritional Values: Calories 150; Carbs 19g; Fat 6.2g; Protein 5.9g

Mushroom Sausages

Serving Size: 12

Cooking Time: 2 hours

Ingredients:

- 6 celery ribs, chopped
- 1 pound no-sugar, beef sausage, chopped
- 2 tablespoons olive oil
- 1/2 pound mushrooms, chopped
- 1/2 cup sunflower seeds, peeled
- 1 cup low-sodium veggie stock
- 1 cup cranberries, dried
- 2 yellow onions, chopped
- 2 garlic cloves, minced
- 1 tablespoon sage, dried
- 1 whole wheat bread loaf, cubed

Directions:

- Heat up a pan with the oil over medium-high heat, add beef, stir and brown for a few minutes.
- Add mushrooms, onion, celery, garlic and sage, stir, cook for a few more minutes and transfer to your slow cooker.
- Add stock, cranberries, sunflower seeds and the bread cubes, cover and cook on High for 2 hours. Stir the whole mix, divide between plates and serve as a side dish.

Nutritional Values: Calories 188; Carbs 8.2g; Fat 13.8g; Protein 7.6g

White Cabbage and Lentils with Relish

Serving Size: 4

Cooking Time: 1 hour 30 minutes

Ingredients:

- 1 medium head of white cabbage, shredded
- 2 cups of boiling water
- Juice from 1 lemon
- Freshly ground black pepper, to taste
- ½ cup of lentils (canned or dried and soaked the night before)
- ½ small cucumber, diced
- 1 tablespoon of dried dill
- 1 cup of fat free Greek yogurt/sour cream

Directions:

- Add the cabbage, water and half the lemon juice to the slow cooker pot. Season generously with freshly ground black pepper.
- Add in enough water until it just covers the cabbage.
- Add the lentils and stir well.
- Set the slow cooker to a heat of LOW and cook for 1½ hours: the dish is ready when most of the prepared water has been actually soaked up.
- While the cabbage is cooking, make the cucumber and dill relish:
- Mix the cucumbers, dill, remaining lemon juice and Greek yogurt and set aside to chill.
- Serve the cabbage with the cucumber and dill relish spooned over the top.

Nutritional Values: Calories 159; Carbs 32g; Fat 1g; Protein 16g

Chapter 4.
Soups and Side Dishes

Basil Zucchini Soup

Serving Size: 4

Cooking Time: 20 minutes

Ingredients:

- 2 tablespoons olive oil
- 3 garlic cloves, minced
- 1 yellow onion, chopped
- 4 zucchinis, cubed
- 4 cups chicken stock
- Zest of 1 lemon, grated
- ½ cup basil, chopped
- Salt and black pepper to the taste

Directions:

- Heat the oil over medium heat in a large saucepan, then add the onion and garlic and simmer, stirring periodically, for 5 minutes.
- Combine the zucchinis with the other ingredients (except the basil), bring to a boil, and cook for 15 minutes over medium heat.
- Add the basil, stir, divide the soup into bowls and serve.

Nutritional Values: Calories 274; Carbs 16.5g; Fat 11.1g; Protein 4.5g

Ham and Bean Soup

Serving Size: 8

Cooking Time: 5 hours

Ingredients:

- ½ (16-ounce) package navy beans
- (14-ounce) cans chicken broth
- 2 cups of water
- 1 cup of carrots, thinly sliced
- 1 cup of onion, finely chopped
- 2 cloves of garlic, sliced
- 1 (14-ounce) can diced tomatoes, with juice
- ½ teaspoon of black pepper
- 1 ½ teaspoons of seasoned salt
- 1 cup of green cabbage, finely chopped
- 1 (5-ounce) can smoked ground ham

Directions:

- Wash navy beans according to package directions.
- Bring one quart of the prepared water to a boil in a pot that is big enough to hold it. Turn off the heat, add the beans, cover, and let them rest for one hour so that they may soften up. After that, drain them.
- Add the ham, cabbage, broth, water, carrots, onion, garlic, tomatoes, pepper, seasoned salt, and seasoned salt, along with the seasoning packet. Cook the beans, covered, over a low heat for three to four hours, or until they are extremely soft. Mix it up every so often.
- The beans should be actually mashed with a potato masher until about half of the beans are broken up, and then they should be stirred to combine.

Nutritional Values: Calories 177; Carbs 26g; Fat 2g; Protein 14g

Paprika and Chives Potatoes

Serving Size: 2

Cooking Time: 58 minutes

Ingredients:

- 4 potatoes
- 1 tablespoon olive oil
- 1 celery stalk, chopped
- 2 tomatoes, chopped
- 1 teaspoon sweet paprika
- 2 tablespoons chives, chopped

Directions:

- Situate potatoes on a baking sheet lined with parchment paper bake at 350 degrees F for 1 hour.
- Cool the potatoes down, peel, and cut them into larger cubes.
- Preheat the pan with the oil over medium heat, add the celery and the tomatoes and sauté for 2 minutes.
- Add the potatoes and the rest of the ingredients, toss, cook everything for 6 minutes, divide the mix between plates and serve.

Nutritional Values: Calories 233; Carbs 12.4g; Fat 8.7g; Protein 6.4g

Pesto Broccoli Quinoa

Serving Size: 4

Cooking Time: 30 minutes

Ingredients:

- 2 and ½ cups quinoa
- 4 and ½ cups veggie stock
- A pinch of salt and black pepper
- 2 tablespoons basil pesto
- 2 cups mozzarella cheese, shredded
- 1-pound broccoli florets
- 1/3 cup parmesan, grated
- 2 green onions, chopped

Directions:

- In a baking pan, combine the quinoa with the stock and the rest of the ingredients except the parmesan and the mozzarella and toss.
- Sprinkle the cheese on top and bake everything at 400 degrees F and bake for 30 minutes.
- Divide between plates and serve as a side dish.

Nutritional Values: Calories 181; Carbs 8.6g; Fat 3.4g; Protein 7.6g

Vegetable Panini

Serving Size: 4

Cooking Time: 25 minutes

Ingredients:

- 2 tablespoons olive oil, divided
- ¼ cup onion, diced
- 1 cup zucchini, diced
- 1 ½ cups broccoli, diced
- ¼ teaspoon of oregano
- sea salt & black pepper to taste
- 12 oz. jar roasted red peppers, drained & chopped fine
- 2 tablespoons of parmesan cheese, grated
- 1 cup mozzarella, fresh & sliced
- 2-foot-long whole grain italian loaf, cut into 4 pieces

Directions:

- Heat your oven to 450°F, and then get out a baking sheet. Heat the oven with your baking sheet inside. Get out a bowl and mix your broccoli, zucchini, oregano, pepper, onion, and salt with a tablespoon of olive oil.

- Take out your baking sheet and spray it with nonstick cooking spray. Spread the vegetable mixture over it to roast for five minutes. Stir halfway through.

- Take it from the oven, and add your red pepper, and sprinkle with parmesan cheese. Mix everything. Get out a panini maker or grill pan, placing it over medium-high heat. Heat a tablespoon of oil.

- Spread the bread horizontally on it, but don't cut it all the way through. Fill with the vegetable mix, and then a slice of mozzarella cheese on top.

- Close the sandwich and cook like you would a normal panini. With a press, it should grill for five minutes. For a grill pan, cook for two and a half minutes per side. Repeat for the remaining sandwiches.

Nutritional Values: Calories 352; Carbs 45g; Fat 15g; Protein 16g

30-Day Meal Plan

Day	Breakfast	Lunch	Dinner
1	Cauliflower Based Waffles	Honey Balsamic Salmon and Lemon Asparagus	Bell Peppers and Sausage
2	Brussels Sprouts Delight	Spaghetti Bolognese	Green Bean Casserole
3	Eggs and Veggies	Cashew Chicken Curry	Brown Rice Pilaf with Butternut Squash
4	Zucchini Skilletcakes	Miso Chicken with Sesame	Tangy Chicken Drumsticks
5	Cauliflower Based Waffles	Cashew Chicken Curry	Bell Peppers and Sausage
6	Spiced Oatmeal	Veal Parmesan	Tangy Chicken Drumsticks
7	Brussels Sprouts Delight	Spaghetti Bolognese	Nut-Crusted Chicken Breasts
8	Eggs and Veggies	Cashew Chicken Curry	Brown Rice Pilaf with Butternut Squash
9	Cauliflower Based Waffles	Veal Parmesan	Nut-Crusted Chicken Breasts
10	Zucchini Skilletcakes	Miso Chicken with Sesame	Tangy Chicken Drumsticks
11	Brussels Sprouts Delight	Spaghetti Bolognese	Bell Peppers and Sausage
12	Spiced Oatmeal	Veal Parmesan	Nut-Crusted Chicken Breasts
13	Zucchini Skilletcakes	Cashew Chicken Curry	Green Bean Casserole
14	Cauliflower Based Waffles	Honey Balsamic Salmon and Lemon Asparagus	Bell Peppers and Sausage
15	Brussels Sprouts Delight	Veal Parmesan	Brown Rice Pilaf with Butternut Squash

16	Spiced Oatmeal	Miso Chicken with Sesame	Tangy Chicken Drumsticks
17	Zucchini Skilletcakes	Honey Balsamic Salmon and Lemon Asparagus	Green Bean Casserole
18	Eggs and Veggies	Cashew Chicken Curry	Nut-Crusted Chicken Breasts
19	Brussels Sprouts Delight	Spaghetti Bolognese	Bell Peppers and Sausage
20	Zucchini Skilletcakes	Veal Parmesan	Tangy Chicken Drumsticks
21	Cauliflower Based Waffles	Cashew Chicken Curry	Brown Rice Pilaf with Butternut Squash
22	Spiced Oatmeal	Miso Chicken with Sesame	Tangy Chicken Drumsticks
23	Eggs and Veggies	Honey Balsamic Salmon and Lemon Asparagus	Green Bean Casserole
24	Cauliflower Based Waffles	Spaghetti Bolognese	Nut-Crusted Chicken Breasts
25	Zucchini Skilletcakes	Miso Chicken with Sesame	Brown Rice Pilaf with Butternut Squash
26	Eggs and Veggies	Veal Parmesan	Nut-Crusted Chicken Breasts
27	Spiced Oatmeal	Honey Balsamic Salmon and Lemon Asparagus	Green Bean Casserole
28	Brussels Sprouts Delight	Spaghetti Bolognese	Bell Peppers and Sausage
29	Spiced Oatmeal	Miso Chicken with Sesame	Brown Rice Pilaf with Butternut Squash
30	Eggs and Veggies	Honey Balsamic Salmon and Lemon Asparagus	Green Bean Casserole

BOOK 5.
DR. NOWZARADAN'S LOW CARB HIGH PROTEIN RECIPES

Introduction

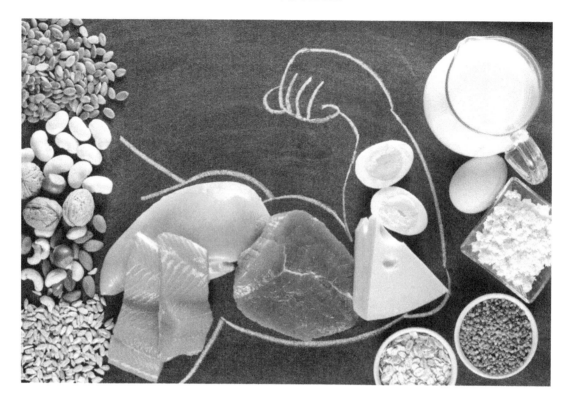

This diet is based on a low-carbohydrate, high-protein diet. Foods that are allowed include egg whites, low-fat dairy, seeds, and low-calorie vegetables. Fruits that have a low glycemic index are also recommended.

In addition, patients are encouraged to reduce their calorie intake in order to lose weight before their surgery. For this reason, the diet can be restrictive. The diet focuses on whole foods and discourages the consumption of processed meats and whole-wheat breads. In addition, the diet requires patients to avoid sweets, snacks, and other high-calorie foods.

The diet can be helpful if the patient can follow it closely. However, if they have other health conditions, such as diabetes or kidney disease, then the diet is not right for them. In fact, patients with diabetes should not even eat sugary snacks, such as sweetened fruit or pudding.

A few foods that are excluded from the diet are white and brown rice, fried meats, candy, fruit juices, and cereal. The Nowzaradan's low-calorie, high-protein diet plan is ideal for those who are preparing for weight loss surgery. This diet is meant to help prepare people for their surgery and encourage them to adopt new eating habits. It is important to remember that weight loss surgery is not a permanent solution to obesity, so patients are encouraged to make long-term changes to their diet and lifestyle.

High-protein

Besides the fact that he is a physician with a lot of weight loss experience, he is also a very popular doctor on television. His popular show My 600 lb Life documents the weight loss journeys of overweight people. The diet is touted as the best diet for morbidly obese patients.

However, the diet can make a significant difference to your quality of life. If you're a morbidly obese patient, it might just be the thing to save your life.

The diet is also a great way to find out if you're actually capable of losing weight. The program features a 12oo-calorie menu, with a variety of foods from protein to fruit. The diet is also designed to lower the risk of surgical complications.

In addition to the standard fare of protein and fruits, the diet also features other dietary staples, including low-fat dairy, low-fat deli meats, low-fat meats, and low-fat vegetables. The diet's other perks include portion control and timed eating.

The diet is also a good way to see if you're ready to make the decision to have bariatric surgery. While the diet is not a cure-all, it's certainly a start. Having a doctor's support is also key to your success.

The diet also has a few drawbacks, such as the dreaded calorie count. Fortunately, the diet's other perks, like portion control and timed eating, are also worth it. You'll also be happy to know that you won't have to worry about putting back on all the weight you've lost.

Chapter 1.
Breakfast

Chicken Souvlaki

Serving Size: 4

Cooking Time: 5 minutes

Ingredients:

- 4 pieces (6-inch) pitas, cut into halves
- 2 cups roasted chicken breast skinless, and sliced
- 1/4 cup red onion, thinly sliced
- 1/2 teaspoon dried oregano
- 1/2 cup Greek yogurt, plain
- 1/2 cup plum tomato, chopped
- 1/2 cup cucumber, peeled, chopped
- 1/2 cup (2 ounces) feta cheese, crumbled
- 1 tablespoon olive oil, extra-virgin, divided
- 1 tablespoon fresh dill, chopped
- 1 cup iceberg lettuce, shredded
- 1 1/4 teaspoons minced garlic, bottled, divided

Directions:

- In a large-sized mixing bowl, combine the 1 teaspoon of the olive oil, yogurt, , and 1/4 teaspoon of the garlic and cheese.
- Oil and heat the pan to cook the chicken, 1 teaspoon garlic and the oregano.
- Put 1/4 cup chicken into each pita halves. Top with 2 tablespoons yogurt mix, 2 tablespoons lettuce,1 tablespoon tomato, and 1 tablespoon cucumber. Divide the onion between the pita halves.

Nutritional Values: Calories 414; Carbs 38g; Fat 6.4g; Protein 32.3g

Eggs Florentine

Serving Size: 1

Cooking Time: 8 minutes

Ingredients:

- 2 large eggs (2 large)
- extra virgin olive oil (1 tbsp., unfiltered)
- Egg Fast Alfredo Sauce (5 tbsp.)
- Organic Parmigiano Reggiano Wedge (1 tbsp., divided)
- organic baby spinach (3 grams)
- red pepper flakes (1 pinch)

Directions:

- Place the oven rack in the top groove of the oven closest to the broiler. Preheat the broiler to high heat.
- Place the olive oil in a nonstick pan and heat over medium high heat until hot but not smoking.
- Using a medium burner, gently cook the eggs until the egg whites are opaque but the yolks are still runny. This will take around 4 minutes. Do not flip the eggs over.
- While you're waiting, start preparing the dish. Pour a little amount of the prepared olive oil into each casserole dish or sprinkle with nonstick cooking spray (olive oil).
- Half of the Alfredo sauce should be put on the bottom of the casserole dish. Slide the half-done egg on top of the sauce with care. Over the eggs, spread some of the remaining Alfredo sauce and half of the parmesan Parmesan.
- Place the casserole in the broiler for approximately about 2-3 minutes, or until the eggs have formed and the top is bubbling with golden spots, depending on your preference.
- Finish by topping with thinly sliced (julienne) baby spinach leaves, any remaining Parmesan cheese, and a sprinkle of red pepper flakes after removing from the broiler. Instantaneous service is provided.

Nutritional Values: Calories 129; Carbs 3g; Fat 3g; Protein 29g

Ground Pork Wonton Ravioli

Serving Size: 6

Cooking Time: 30 minutes

Ingredients:

- 8 ounces of ground pork
- 4 ounces of shrimp
- 1 green onion, finely chopped
- 2 garlic cloves, minced
- 1-inch fresh ginger root, peeled and minced
- 1 egg white
- 1 teaspoon of cornstarch
- 1 teaspoon of garlic chili paste
- Juice of ¼ of a lemon
- 1 tablespoon of low-sodium soy sauce
- Pinch of salt and black pepper
- 1 tablespoon of ground shiitake mushrooms dried
- 2 drops of toasted sesame oil
- 3 large Savoy cabbage leaves, shredded fine
- 36 round wonton wrappers

Directions:

- Place all ingredients except the cabbage and wrappers into a food processor and grind to form a paste. Fold in shredded cabbage.
- Place a wonton wrapper on cutting board or counter. Put 1 tablespoon of prepared filling in the center of wonton. Brush cold water on edges of the wonton and cover with a second wonton. Carefully remove all air and seal edges. Poach in water or stock until they float.

Nutritional Values: Calories 130; Carbs 6g; Fat 3g; Protein 5g

Onion Frittata

Serving Size: 4

Cooking Time: 2 hours

Ingredients:

- A pinch of white pepper
- 1 tablespoon olive oil
- ½ cup yellow onion, chopped
- 1 cup low-fat cheese, shredded
- 1 cup baby spinach leaves
- 1 tomato, chopped
- 3 egg whites
- 3 eggs
- 2 tablespoon low-fat milk
- A pinch of black pepper

Directions:

- In a bowl, mix the eggs with the egg whites, milk, white and black pepper, spinach and tomato and stir.
- Grease the slow cooker with the oil, pour eggs mix, spread the cheese on top, cover and cook on Low for 2 hours.
- Slice the frittata, divide between plates and serve.

Nutritional Values: Calories 217; Carbs 3.4g; Fat 16.3g; Protein 14.7g

Veggie Quiche Muffins

Serving Size: 12

Cooking Time: 50 minutes

Ingredients:

- Cheddar (3⁄4 cup, low-fat, shredded)
- Green Onion (1 cup, chopped)
- Broccoli (1 cup, chopped)
- Tomatoes (1 cup, diced)
- Milk (2 cups, non-fat)
- Eggs (4)
- Pancake mix (1 cup)
- Oregano (1 tsp.)
- Salt (1⁄2 tsp.)
- Pepper (1⁄2 tsp.)

Directions:

- Preheat your oven to a heat of 375 degrees Fahrenheit and gently coat a 12-cup muffin tray with cooking oil before starting.
- Fill the muffin cups with the tomatoes, broccoli, onions, and cheddar cheese. Bake for 20 minutes at 350 degrees. In a medium-sized mixing bowl, add the other ingredients and whisk until well combined. Pour the mixture equally over the vegetables.
- Set your preheated oven to bake for about 40 minutes, or until the top is golden brown.
- Allow for a little cooling period (approximately 5 minutes) before serving. Enjoy!

Nutritional Values: Calories 112; Carbs 2.9g; Fat 3.2g; Protein 5.1g

Chapter 2.
Lunch

Chicken Calzone

Serving Size: 12

Cooking Time: 1 hour

Ingredients:

- 2 eggs
- 1 keto pizza crust
- ½ cup parmesan, grated
- 1 pound chicken breasts, skinless, boneless and each sliced in halves
- ½ cup keto marinara sauce
- 1 teaspoon Italian seasoning
- 1 teaspoon onion powder
- 1 teaspoon garlic powder
- Salt and black pepper to the taste
- ¼ cup flaxseed, ground
- 8 ounces provolone cheese

Directions:

- In a bowl, mix Italian seasoning with onion powder, garlic powder, salt, pepper, flaxseed and parmesan and stir well.
- In another bowl, mix eggs with a pinch of salt and pepper and whisk well.
- Dip chicken pieces in eggs and then in seasoning mix, place all pieces on a lined baking sheet and bake in the oven at 350 degrees F for 30 minutes.
- Put pizza crust dough on a lined baking sheet and spread half of the provolone cheese on half. Take chicken out of the oven, chop and spread over provolone cheese. Add marinara sauce and then the rest of the cheese.
- Cover all these with the other half of the dough and shape your calzone.
- Seal its edges, introduce in the oven at 350 degrees F and bake for 20 minuets more.
- Leave calzone to cool down before slicing and serving. Enjoy!

Nutritional Values: Calories 340; Fat 8g; Carbohydrates 6g; Protein 20g

Chicken Cordon Bleu

Serving Size: 4

Cooking Time: 2 hours

Ingredients:

- 2 boneless, skinless chicken breasts, butterflied
- 4 deli slices ham
- 4 deli slices Swiss cheese
- ½ cup flour
- 1 egg
- 1 cup bread crumbs

Directions:

- Preheat the water bath to 140°F. Lay slices of ham on top of butterflied chicken breasts, then lay cheese on top of ham.
- Trim excess. Roll up chicken breasts with the ham and cheese on the inside.
- Place prepared chicken breasts inside the bag. Seal tightly and place in water bath. Cook 1 ½ hours.
- When chicken is done, remove carefully from wrapper and pat dry. Dredge each prepared piece in flour, then dip in egg, followed by the breadcrumbs. Preheat your air fryer to 350°F.
- Air Fry chicken until golden brown on all sides.
- Remove to paper towel to drain. Cut breasts in halves, then serve.

Nutritional Values: Calories 448; Carbs 34.2g; Fat 26g; Protein 46.2g

Crispy Pollock and Gazpacho

Serving Size: 3

Cooking Time: 15 minutes

Ingredients:

- 85 g whole-wheat bread, torn into chunks
- 4 tablespoons olive oil
- 4 pieces Pollock fillets, skinless
- 4 large tomatoes, cut into chunks
- 3/4 cucumber, cut into chunks
- 2 tablespoons sherry vinegar
- 2 garlic cloves, crushed
- 1/2 red onion, thinly sliced
- 1 yellow pepper, deseeded, cut into chunks

Directions:

- Preheat the oven to 200C, gas to 6, or fan to 180C.
- Over a baking tray, scatter the chunks of bread. Toss with 1 tablespoon of the prepared olive oil and bake for about 10 minutes, or until golden and crispy.
- Meanwhile, mix the cucumber, tomatoes, onion, pepper, crushed garlic, sherry vinegar, and 2 tablespoons of the olive oil; season well.
- Heat a non-stick large frying pan. Add the remaining prepared 1 tablespoon of the olive oil and heat. When the prepared oil is already hot, add the fish; cook for about 4 minutes or until golden. Flip the fillet; cook for additional 1 to 2 minutes or until the fish cooked through.
- In a mixing bowl, quickly toss the salad and the croutons; divide among 4 plates and then serve with the fish.

Nutritional Values: Calories 296; Carbs 19g; Fat 13g; Protein 27g

Thyme Ginger Garlic Beef

Serving Size: 2

Cooking Time: 45 minutes

Ingredients:

- 1 lb beef roast
- 2 whole cloves
- 1/2 teaspoon ginger, grated
- 1/2 cup beef stock
- 1/2 teaspoon garlic powder
- 1/2 teaspoon thyme
- 1/4 teaspoon pepper
- 1/4 teaspoon salt

Directions:

- Mix together ginger, cloves, thyme, garlic powder, pepper, and salt and rub over beef.
- Place meat into the instant pot. Pour stock around the meat.
- Seal pot with cover lid and cook on high for 45 minutes.
- Once done, release pressure using quick release. Remove lid.
- Shred meat using a fork and serve.

Nutritional Values: Calories 452; Carbs 5.2g; Fat 15.7g; Protein 70.1g

Zucchini and Lemon Herb Salmon

Serving Size: 4

Cooking Time: 20 minutes

Ingredients:

- 2 tablespoon olive oil
- 4 chopped zucchinis
- 2 tablespoon lemon juice
- 2 tablespoon agave nectar
- 2 garlic cloves, minced
- 1 tablespoon Dijon mustard
- ½ teaspoon oregano, dried
- ½ teaspoon dill, dried
- ¼ teaspoon rosemary, dried
- ¼ teaspoon thyme, dried
- 4 salmon fillets
- 2 tablespoon parsley leaves, chopped
- Ground black pepper and kosher salt to taste

Directions:

- Preheat your oven to 400°F. Apply cooking spray on your baking sheet lightly.
- Whisk together the lemon juice, brown sugar, dill, garlic, Dijon, rosemary, thyme, and oregano in a bowl. Season with pepper and salt to taste. Set aside.
- Keep the zucchini on your baking sheet in one single layer.
- Drizzle some olive oil. Season with pepper and salt.
- Add the fish in one layer. Brush each fillet with your herb mix.
- Keep in the oven. Cook for 17 minutes. Garnish with parsley and serve.

Nutritional Values: Calories 355; Carbs 15g; Fat 19g; Protein 31g

Chapter 3.
Dinner

Asparagus and Lemon Salmon

Serving Size: 3

Cooking Time: 15 minutes

Ingredients:

- 2 salmon fillets, 6 ounces each, skin on
- Sunflower seeds to taste
- 1 pound asparagus, trimmed
- 2 cloves garlic, minced
- 3 tablespoons almond butter
- ¼ cup cashew cheese

Directions:

- Preheat your oven to 400 degrees F.
- Line a baking sheet with oil.
- Take a kitchen towel and pat your salmon dry, season as needed.
- Put salmon onto the baking sheet and arrange asparagus around it.
- Place a pan over medium heat and melt almond butter.
- Add garlic and cook for 3 minutes until garlic browns slightly.
- Drizzle sauce over salmon.
- Sprinkle salmon with cheese and bake for 12 minutes until salmon looks cooked all the way and is flaky.
- Serve and enjoy!

Nutritional Values: Calories 434; Carbs 6g; Fat 26g; Protein 42g

Balsamic Steaks

Serving Size: 4

Cooking Time: 15 minutes

Ingredients:

- 1 pound beef steaks, cut into 4 sliced
- 2 tablespoons olive oil
- Salt and black pepper to the taste
- ¼ cup balsamic vinegar
- 2 garlic cloves, minced
- 1 teaspoon red pepper flakes
- 1 teaspoon garlic powder
- 2 shallots, chopped
- 1 tablespoon chives, chopped

Directions:

- Heat up a pan with the oil over medium heat, add the garlic, shallots, pepper flakes and garlic powder, stir and sauté for 5 minutes.
- Add the steaks and the other ingredients, cook them for 5 minutes on each side, divide between plates and serve.

Nutritional Values: Calories 435; Carbs 10g; Fat 23g; Protein 35g

Crab Mushrooms

Serving Size: 5

Cooking Time: 15 minutes

Ingredients:

- 7 oz. crab meat
- 10 oz. white mushrooms
- ½ teaspoon salt
- ¼ cup fish stock
- 1 teaspoon butter
- ¼ teaspoon ground coriander
- 1 teaspoon dried cilantro
- 1 teaspoon butter

Directions:

- Chop the crab meat and sprinkle it with the salt and dried cilantro.
- Mix the crab meat carefully. Preheat the air fryer to 400 F.
- Chop the white mushrooms and combine them with the crab meat.
- After this, add the fish stock, ground coriander, and butter.
- Transfer the side dish mixture in the air fryer basket tray.
- Stir it gently with the help of the plastic spatula.
- Cook the side dish for 5 minutes.
- When the time is over – let the dish rest for 5 minutes.
- Then serve it. Enjoy!

Nutritional Values: Calories 356; Carbs 2.6g; Fat 1.7g; Protein 7g

Seared Scallops and Roasted Grapes

Serving Size: 4

Cooking Time: 10 minutes

Ingredients:

- 1 pound scallops
- 3 tablespoons olive oil
- 1 shallot, chopped
- 3 garlic cloves, minced
- 2 cups spinach
- 1 cup chicken stock
- 1 romanesco lettuce head
- 1 and ½ cups red grapes, cut in halves
- ¼ cup walnuts, toasted and chopped
- 1 tablespoon ghee
- Salt and black pepper to the taste

Directions:

- Put romanesco in your food processor, blend and transfer to a bowl.
- Heat up a large-sized pan with 2 tablespoons oil over medium high heat, add shallot and garlic, stir and cook for 1 minute.
- Add romanesco, spinach and 1 cup stock, stir, cook for 3 minutes, blend using an immersion blender and take off heat.
- Heat up another pan with 1 tablespoon oil and the ghee over medium high heat, add scallops, season with salt and pepper, cook for 2 minutes, flip and sear for 1 minute more.
- Divide romanesco mix on plates, add scallops on the side, top with walnuts and grapes and serve. Enjoy!

Nutritional Values: Calories 300; Fat 12g; Carbohydrates 6g; Protein 20g

Turnip Greens and Artichoke Chicken

Serving Size: 4

Cooking Time: 40 minutes

Ingredients:

- 4 oz canned artichoke heart chopped
- 4 oz cream cheese
- 2 chicken breasts cut
- 1 cup turnip greens
- 1/4 cup Pecorino cheese, grated
- 1/2 tablespoon onion powder
- 1/2 tablespoon garlic powder
- Black pepper and salt to taste
- 2 oz Monterrey Jack Shredded

Directions:

- Prepare a large-sized baking dish by covering it with parchment paper and placing the chicken pieces in the bottom. Sprinkle salt and pepper on top. Bake to 350 F and bake for 20 to 25 minutes.
- In a mixing bowl, mix the other ingredients and mix thoroughly. Take the cooked chicken out of the oven, and place it on top of the artichokes. Sprinkle the dish with Monterrey cheese, and cook for five more minutes. Serve warm.

Nutritional Values: Calories 373; Carbs 6.2g; Fat 29g; Protein 31g

Chapter 3.
Snacks

Cinnamon Stuffed Peaches

Serving Size: 4

Cooking Time: 15 minutes

Ingredients:

- 4 peaches, pitted, halved
- 2 tablespoons ricotta cheese
- 2 tablespoons of liquid honey
- ¾ cup of water
- ½ teaspoon vanilla extract
- ¾ teaspoon ground cinnamon
- 1 tablespoon of almonds, sliced
- ¾ teaspoon saffron

Directions:

- Pour water in the saucepan and bring to boil.
- Add vanilla extract, saffron, ground cinnamon, and liquid honey.
- Cook the liquid until the honey is melted.
- Then remove it from the heat.
- Put the halved peaches in the hot honey liquid.
- Meanwhile, make the filling: mix up together ricotta cheese, vanilla extract, and sliced almonds.
- Remove the peaches from the honey liquid and arrange them on the plate. Fill 4 peach halves with ricotta filling and cover them with remaining peach halves.
- Sprinkle the cooked dessert with liquid honey mixture gently.

Nutritional Values: Calories 213; Fat 1.4g; Carbohydrates 23.9g; Protein 1.9g

Mashed Beets

Serving Size: 4

Cooking Time: 40 minutes

Ingredients:

- 4 whole beets, trimmed and peeled
- 1 tablespoon of olive oil
- ⅓ cup of water
- 1 tablespoon of honey
- 2 tablespoons of cider vinegar
- ½ teaspoon of garlic powder
- Juice of 1 lemon
- Freshly ground pepper, to taste
- 2 tablespoons of fat free Greek yogurt

Directions:

- Combine the beets with the other ingredients and arrange them in the slow cooker pot (reserve the yogurt).
- Set the slow cooker to LOW until the beets are soft enough to mash.
- Swirl through the Greek yogurt and mash until smooth.
- Serve as a delicious snack or with your favorite high protein main dish.

Nutritional Values: Calories 275; Carbs 11g; Fat 4g; Protein 2g

Pork Beef Bean Nachos

Serving Size: 10

Cooking Time: 40 minutes

Ingredients:

- 1 package beef jerky
- 4 cans black beans, drained and rinsed
- 6 bacon strips, crumbled
- 3 pounds pork spareribs
- 1 cup chopped onion
- 4 teaspoons minced garlic
- 4 cups divided beef broth
- optional toppings such as cheddar, sour cream, green onions, jalapeno slices
- 1 teaspoon crushed red pepper flakes

Directions:

- Pulse jerky in processor till ground, working in batches, put the ribs in the instant pot, topping with half jerky, two beans, ½ cup onion, three pieces of bacon, 2 teaspoons garlic, 2 cups broth, and half teaspoon red pepper flakes. Cook on high for forty minutes.
- Let it natural pressure release for approximately about 10 minutes, then quick release what's next, and do the same with the second batch.
- Discard bones, and shred meat and then sauté it, and strain the mixture, and then discard juice and serve with chips and your desired toppings.

Nutritional Values: Calories 269; Carbs 27g; Fat 24g; Protein 33g

Shrimps Ceviche

Serving Size: 8

Cooking Time: 6 minutes

Ingredients:

- ¼ pound shrimp, peeled, deveined and chopped
- Zest and juice of 2 limes
- Zest and juice of 2 lemons
- 2 teaspoons cumin, ground
- 2 tablespoons olive oil
- 1 cup tomato, chopped
- ½ cup red onion, chopped
- 2 tablespoons garlic, minced
- 1 Serrano chili pepper, chopped
- 1 cup black beans, canned and drained
- 1 cup cucumber, chopped
- ¼ cup cilantro, chopped

Directions:

- In a bowl, mix lime juice and lemon juice with shrimp, toss well, cover and keep in the fridge for 3 hours.
- Heat up a pan with the oil over medium high heat, add shrimp and citrus juices, cook for 2 minutes on each side and transfer everything to a bowl.
- Add lime and lemon zest, cumin, tomato, onion, garlic, chili pepper, cucumber, black beans and cilantro, toss well and serve with some tortilla chips on the side.

Nutritional Values: Calories 100; Carbs 10g; Fat 3g; Protein 5g

Spiced Tea Pudding

Serving Size: 3

Cooking Time: 10 minutes

Ingredients:

- ½ cup coconut flakes
- ½ teaspoon cloves
- 1(½) cup berries
- 1 can coconut milk
- 1 cup almond milk
- 1 tablespoon chia seeds
- 1 tablespoon ground cinnamon
- 1 tablespoon raw honey
- 1 teaspoon allspice
- 1 teaspoon cardamom
- 1 teaspoon green tea powder
- 1 teaspoon nutmeg
- ½ tablespoon pumpkin seeds
- 1 teaspoon ground ginger

Directions:

- In your blender, puree tea powder with coconut milk, almond milk, cinnamon, coconut flakes, nutmeg, allspice, cloves, honey, cardamom, and ginger split into bowls.
- Heat a pan on moderate heat, put in berries until bubbling, then move to your blender and pulse well. Split the berries into the bowls with the coconut milk mix. Top with chia seeds and pumpkin seeds before you serve. Enjoy!

Nutritional Values: Calories 150; Fat 6g; Carbohydrates 14g; Protein 8g

Chapter 4.
Soup and Side Dishes
Coconut and Lemongrass Turkey Soup

Serving Size: 5

Cooking Time: 40 minutes

Ingredients:

- 1 teaspoon of finely sliced lemongrass
- 1 teaspoon of ground ginger
- 1 garlic clove, minced
- 1 tablespoon of fresh cilantro, chopped
- 1 tablespoon of dried basil
- Juice of 1 lime
- 1 tablespoon of coconut oil
- 1 cup of diced white onion
- 12 ounces of skinless turkey breast, diced
- ½ cup of low fat chicken broth
- ½ cup of water
- 1 cup of snow peas

Directions:

- Crush the lemongrass, ginger, garlic, cilantro, basil, and lime juice in a mortar and pestle to form a paste. Heat the prepared coconut oil in a skillet over medium-high heat and stir-fry the paste for 1 minute. Add the onions and turkey to the skillet and coat evenly with the paste to brown. Add the broth and water, and gently stir. Remove from the heat, and transfer to the slow cooker. Set the slow cooker to LOW for approximately about 4-6 hours.
- Add the snow peas to the soup 15 minutes before the end of the cooking time. Top with scallions and fresh cilantro if desired.

Nutritional Values: Calories 287; Carbs 9g; Fat 5g; Protein 16g

Margherita Slices

Serving Size: 4

Cooking Time: 15 minutes

Ingredients:

- 1 tomato, cut into 8 slices
- 1 clove garlic, halved
- 1 tablespoon of olive oil
- ¼ teaspoon of oregano
- 1 cup mozzarella, fresh & sliced
- ¼ cup basil leaves, fresh, tron & lightly packed
- sea salt & black pepper to taste
- 2 hoagie rolls, 6 inches each

Directions:

- Start by heating your oven broiler to high. Your rack should be four inches under the heating element.
- Lay the sliced bread on a rimmed baking pan. Broil for a minute. Your bread should be toasted lightly. Brush each one down with oil and rub your garlic over each half.
- Place the bread back on your baking sheet. Distribute the tomato slices on each one, and then sprinkle with oregano and cheese.
- Bake for one to two minutes, but check it after a minute. Your cheese should be melted.
- Top with basil and pepper before serving.

Nutritional Values: Calories 297; Carbs 38g; Fat 11g; Protein 12g

Smoked Salmon, Avocado, and Cucumber Bites

Serving Size: 1

Cooking Time: 0 minutes

Ingredients:

- 1/2 cucumber, medium size
- 3 oz Smoked salmon
- 1/2 avocado, peeled, and remove the pit
- 1/2 tbsp Lime juice
- Salt and ground black pepper for garnish
- Chopped fresh chives for serving

Directions:

- Cut the cucumber into 1/4th inch of thickness. Place them on a plate.
- In a bowl, add lime juice and avocado, mash with a fork until smooth.
- On each cucumber slice, spread the avocado mixture. On top, place a piece of smoked salmon.
- Add another slice of cucumber on top.
- Sprinkle salt and freshly ground black pepper on top.
- Serve right away with fresh chives.

Nutritional Values: Calories 243; Carbs 29.4g; Fat 15.4g; Protein 13.8g

Spicy Carrot and Lime Soup

Serving Size: 2

Cooking Time: 7-8 hours

Ingredients:

- 1 teaspoon of mustard seeds, crushed
- 1 teaspoon of fennel seeds, crushed
- 1 tablespoon of ground ginger
- 4 medium carrots, peeled and chopped
- 1 cup of diced red onion
- 1 lime, zest and juice
- 2 cups of water
- 1 tablespoon of fresh oregano, chopped
- ½ cup of fat free Greek yogurt
- Freshly ground black pepper, to taste

Directions:

- Heat a non-stick skillet over medium-high heat. Add the crushed mustard seeds and fennel seeds and stir-fry for a minute. Add the ground ginger and cook for another minute.
- Add the carrots, onions, and lime juice and cook until the vegetables are softened, about 5 minutes. Remove from the heat and transfer to the slow cooker pot.
- Add the water, lime zest and juice, and fresh oregano to the pot.
- Set the slow cooker to LOW for approximately about 7-8 hours or HIGH for 3-4 hours.
- Serve with ¼ cup of Greek yogurt swirled through and black pepper to taste.

Nutritional Values: Calories 224; Carbs 32g; Fat 1g; Protein 16g

White Bean and Kale Soup with Chicken

Serving Size: 6

Cooking Time: 30 minutes

Ingredients:

- Sea salt + black pepper
- 3 cups kale
- 1 15-oz can white beans
- 2 cups chicken
- 1 strip bacon
- 4 cloves garlic
- 8 cups broth
- 1 cup white onion
- 1 tablespoon avocado oil

Directions:

- Over moderate flame, heat a large pan or casserole dish. Once the pan is warmed, add the bacon or oil. Allow for two minutes of cooking time, stirring occasionally.
- Cook, stirring periodically, for 4-5 minutes, or until onions becomes transparent and citrusy.
- Then add garlic and cook for another 2-3 minutes. Carry to a boil the broth, completely soaked white beans and meat.
- To blend the flavors, cook for ten minutes. After that, sprinkle with salt and pepper. Insert the kale over the last few minutes before serving. Serve instantly.

Nutritional Values: Calories 280; Carbs 7.4g; Fat 12.1g; Protein 34g

30-Day Meal Plan

Day	Breakfast	Lunch	Dinner
1	Ground Pork Wonton Ravioli	Chicken Cordon Bleu	Balsamic Steaks
2	Chicken Souvlaki	Crispy Pollock and Gazpacho	Asparagus and Lemon Salmon
3	Eggs Florentine	Zucchini and Lemon Herb Salmon	Seared Scallops and Roasted Grapes
4	Onion Frittata	Thyme Ginger Garlic Beef	Crab Mushrooms
5	Chicken Souvlaki	Chicken Calzone	Balsamic Steaks
6	Ground Pork Wonton Ravioli	Crispy Pollock and Gazpacho	Turnip Greens and Artichoke Chicken
7	Onion Frittata	Chicken Cordon Bleu	Seared Scallops and Roasted Grapes
8	Chicken Souvlaki	Thyme Ginger Garlic Beef	Balsamic Steaks
9	Veggie Quiche Muffins	Crispy Pollock and Gazpacho	Crab Mushrooms
10	Ground Pork Wonton Ravioli	Thyme Ginger Garlic Beef	Turnip Greens and Artichoke Chicken
11	Veggie Quiche Muffins	Chicken Cordon Bleu	Asparagus and Lemon Salmon
12	Eggs Florentine	Zucchini and Lemon Herb Salmon	Seared Scallops and Roasted Grapes
13	Onion Frittata	Crispy Pollock and Gazpacho	Balsamic Steaks
14	Veggie Quiche Muffins	Chicken Calzone	Turnip Greens and Artichoke Chicken
15	Chicken Souvlaki	Thyme Ginger Garlic Beef	Asparagus and Lemon Salmon

16	Eggs Florentine	Chicken Calzone	Crab Mushrooms
17	Onion Frittata	Chicken Cordon Bleu	Seared Scallops and Roasted Grapes
18	Chicken Souvlaki	Zucchini and Lemon Herb Salmon	Asparagus and Lemon Salmon
19	Ground Pork Wonton Ravioli	Crispy Pollock and Gazpacho	Balsamic Steaks
20	Veggie Quiche Muffins	Zucchini and Lemon Herb Salmon	Turnip Greens and Artichoke Chicken
21	Eggs Florentine	Chicken Calzone	Seared Scallops and Roasted Grapes
22	Onion Frittata	Thyme Ginger Garlic Beef	Turnip Greens and Artichoke Chicken
23	Ground Pork Wonton Ravioli	Chicken Cordon Bleu	Balsamic Steaks
24	Veggie Quiche Muffins	Zucchini and Lemon Herb Salmon	Crab Mushrooms
25	Eggs Florentine	Thyme Ginger Garlic Beef	Seared Scallops and Roasted Grapes
26	Onion Frittata	Chicken Calzone	Asparagus and Lemon Salmon
27	Chicken Souvlaki	Crispy Pollock and Gazpacho	Crab Mushrooms
28	Veggie Quiche Muffins	Zucchini and Lemon Herb Salmon	Turnip Greens and Artichoke Chicken
29	Ground Pork Wonton Ravioli	Chicken Calzone	Crab Mushrooms
30	Eggs Florentine	Chicken Cordon Bleu	Asparagus and Lemon Salmon

BOOK 6.
BONUS: LOW-CALORIE KETO RECIPES

Introduction

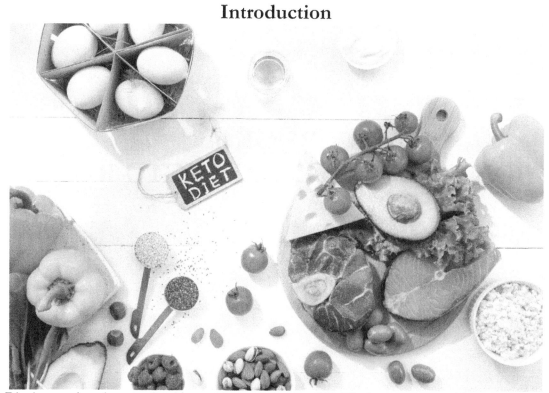

Keto Diet is very clear that one should eat as few carbs as possible. The best answer to this question is that the viable limits for carbs should be between 30 to 100 grams per day. Eating more than 100 grams per day will affect Ketosis.

If you are sure that what you are eating is keto-friendly, there is no need to track your macros. In short, you should not concern yourself with tracking macros if you are eating all foods listed as keto foods. However, you are supposed to track macros if you want to stray from keto foods for a snack or one meal.

Even as the Keto diet may be self-sufficient in providing the body with the required nutrients, supplements can be taken to boost certain deficiencies. However, supplements should be taken with prior consultation and approval of a dietician. Note that an abnormal intake of some supplements can cause enormous effects on the body.

Scientifically, your body can survive without consuming any dietary carbohydrates. Therefore, it is not unhealthy to forgo carbs and instead eat more fat with some protein. These two macros can healthily substitute for carbs. Remember that the main use of carbs in the body is energy production, which can be replaced by Ketosis (use of fats for energy production).

You must have heard that Ketosis is dangerous, especially to keto beginners. Well, it is not dangerous! One may just develop minor systems caused by the keto flu as the body becomes adapted to the Keto Diet. For some people, the flu is usually gone by the end of the first week. However, if the flu prolongs, it cannot go for more than three weeks.

Some people experience short-lived irritability, frequent urination, dehydration, and keto flu. After a short period, the body gets used to a low-carb and high-fat intake.

The only thing you should actually do is reduce your alcohol intake and know the type of alcohol to consume. Do not forget that most alcoholic drinks are very rich in carbs and unfriendly to the Keto Diet. The best option for you is pure spirits in moderate quantities. In addition, do not mix spirits with soda or fruit juices because the net effect will be adding to your carb intake.

The Keto Diet is not for everyone. It is better for people who want to lose weight, improve cognitive function, reduce risks of certain diseases, and enhance endurance, among other personal goals.

Chapter 1.
The Keto Diet

The ideas behind the ketogenic diet are not new. This diet plan was actually created many years ago as a cure for epilepsy in younger children. There are even a few popular diets that are modeled after the ketogenic diet, such as the Paleo diet, the South Beach diet and the Atkins diet. While these diet plans are not exactly the same as the ketogenic diet, they use some of the same basic ideas to help their followers to lose weight

The ketogenic diet is one of the most effective ways for you to lose weight. It allows you to eat foods that will fill you up, without having to worry about gaining weight. You will eat fewer calories, but the foods that you are choosing will help to speed up fat loss, rather than stop it

Let's start from the beginning. A ketogenic diet is going to be a diet that will force the body into ketosis. In ketosis, the body is going to learn how to burn fats, rather than carbs, as energy

In a typical American diet, as well as in other diet plans that don't often work, your body is used to working with carbs for energy. The body likes to use carbs because they are easy to convert into energy, but they are not very efficient

We take in a lot of carbs in a traditional diet. Between eating pastas, breads, pizzas, and even fruits and vegetables, there are carbs around us all the time. These provide us with a nice source of energy through the day, but it is often a high followed by a big crash

When we eat the carbs, we feel good for a little bit. The body has a new source of energy and is ready to go. But the carbs are going to be converted into sugars in the body, which can be extra bad if you are also eating a lot of bad sugars

The insulin will come and take care of the carbs and use them in the cells. But these carbs are usually burnt up before we have used anywhere near the amount of calories that came with them.

The result is that we start to feel tired and sluggish. This usually happens within a few hours. And our bodies start to crave more carbs in the hopes of increasing our energy some more and helping us to get through the day. This is a vicious cycle; the more carbs we eat, the more we need to help keep us energized and we gain weight and belly fat in the process

The ketogenic diet is going to try and change this. Instead of following a diet that either leads you to feeling deprived or leads you to failing, it is going to provide you with the foods and tools that you need to get out of this vicious cycle and start seeing some weight loss results

When you go on the ketogenic diet, you will go through the process of ketosis. In ketosis, you are going to make the body start using fats, instead of carbs, for the energy that it needs. To make this happen, you will limit your carb intake to below fifty grams each day (some individuals who really want to enter ketosis quickly will stick with twenty grams or fewer of carbs each day)

Most of your diet is going to focus on healthy fats so that you provide the body with the energy that it needs.

Fats are much more efficient forms of energy than carbs. You will find that foods that are full of good fats will fill you up for a much longer time and can naturally lead you to eating fewer calories

During the first actual few days of the ketogenic diet, you may feel a little bit lethargic and tired because the body is low on energy and hasn't converted over to ketosis yet. But once that happens, which usually takes between two to seven days, you are going to have more energy than you could ever imagine

It is important for you to figure out which macronutrients you are eating on this diet plan. It is not enough to just eat more fats in your diet and call it good. If you are taking in too many carbs, even with the fat intake going up, you are going to end up losing out on this diet. You will never enter into ketosis and will just add more fat and weight to your body

In addition, if you take in the right amount of carbs and protein, but your fat consumption is not high enough, you will have a hard time keeping your levels of energy up. It is hard to consume more fats, especially since we have been hearing about how bad fats are for the body, but on the ketogenic diet, fats are going to be the body's main source of energy. If you are not taking in enough fats, you will not have enough energy to make it through the day

The reason that these macronutrients are so important is because they will help you to enter ketosis and lose weight. How do you know that you are entering ketosis? Some people take a look at how much weight and fat loss they experience, and others want to know for sure. If you are stalled out on weight loss or you are having trouble figuring out if you are staying within the right carb content, you can choose to use ketostix

Ketostix are able to determine how many ketones are being released into the urine. Ketones are only going to be present when you are in ketosis. They are a good way to monitor whether you are eating the right macronutrients or not

Working with the ketogenic diet can be a great way for you to lose weight and to get rid of some of that excess fat that is hanging around the body. It can be hard to stick with for some people because it does have some restrictions and sticking with the macronutrients. But as you get into the ketogenic diet cookbook, you will be able to find some fantastic recipes that will help you to stick with the diet and feel like you are getting to eat the best meals in the world.

Chapter 2.
Keto Recipes

Baked Granola

Serving Size: 4

Cooking Time: 55 minutes

Ingredients:

- ½ cup almonds, chopped
- 1 cup pecans, chopped
- ½ cup walnuts, chopped
- ½ cup coconut, flaked
- ¼ cup flax meal
- ½ cup almond milk
- ¼ cup sunflower seeds
- ¼ cup pepitas
- ½ cup stevia
- ¼ cup ghee, melted
- 1 teaspoon honey
- 1 teaspoon vanilla
- 1 teaspoon cinnamon, ground
- A pinch of salt
- ½ teaspoon nutmeg
- ¼ cup water

Directions:

- In a bowl, mix almonds with pecans, walnuts, coconut, flax meal, milk, sunflower seeds, pepitas, stevia, ghee, honey, vanilla, cinnamon, salt, nutmeg and water and whisk very well.
- Grease a baking sheet with parchment paper, spread granola mix and press well.
- Cover with another piece of parchment paper, introduce in the oven at 250 degrees F and bake for 1 hour.
- Take granola out of the oven, leave aside to cool down, break into pieces and serve.
- Enjoy!

Nutritional Values: Calories 340; Carbs 8g; Fat 32g; Protein 20g

Beef with Kale and Leeks

Serving Size: 4

Cooking Time: 30 minutes

Ingredients:

- 2 tablespoons olive oil
- 1 pound beef stew meat, cubed
- 1 cup kale, torn
- 2 leeks, chopped
- 1 cup tomato passata
- A pinch of salt and black pepper
- 1 tablespoon cilantro, chopped
- 1 teaspoon sweet paprika
- ½ teaspoon rosemary, dried

Directions:

- Heat up a large-sized pan with the oil over medium heat, add the leeks and the meat and brown for 5 minutes.
- Add the rest of the prepared ingredients, bring to a simmer and cook over medium heat for 25 minutes more.
- Divide everything into bowls and serve.

Nutritional Values: Calories 250; Carbs 3g; Fat 5g; Protein 12g

Hot Dog Rolls

Serving Size: 4

Cooking Time: 20 minutes

Ingredients:

- 4 hot dogs
- ¾ cup almond flour.
- 1 egg
- 1 ½ cups shredded mozzarella cheese.
- 2 tablespoon cream cheese; at room temperature
- 1 teaspoon Italian seasoning.
- 1 teaspoon minced garlic

Directions:

- Preheat your oven to 425-Degrees F. In a large microwaveable bowl, combine the mozzarella cheese and cream cheese. Microwave on high for 1 minute. Remove, stir and microwave again for 30 seconds more. The mixture will be very hot.
- Now, add the almond flour, egg, garlic and Italian seasoning to the cheese mixture. Stir to incorporate fully
- With wet hands, divide the dough into four equal pieces. Shape one piece of dough around each hot dog, encasing the hot dog completely
- Place the dough-wrapped hot dogs onto a parchment-lined baking sheet. Use a fork to poke holes into each piece of dough so it doesn't bubble up during cooking. Put the prepared baking sheet into the preheated oven. Bake for 7 to 8 minutes.
- Remove the tray from the oven. Check for bubbles {prick with a fork, if formed}. Turn the dogs over. Return to the oven for another 6 to 7 minutes.
- Remove the sheet from the oven. Cool the hot dog rolls for 3 to 5 minutes before serving.

Nutritional Values: Calories 435; Carbs 7.6g; Fat 34.7g; Protein 18.6g

Lamb with Fennel and Figs

Serving Size: 4

Cooking Time: 40 minutes

Ingredients:

- 12 ounces lamb racks
- 2 fennel bulbs, sliced
- Salt and black pepper to the taste
- 2 tablespoons olive oil
- 4 figs, cut in halves
- 1/8 cup apple cider vinegar
- 1 tablespoon swerve

Directions:

- In a bowl, mix fennel with figs, vinegar, swerve and oil, toss to coat well and transfer to a baking dish.
- Season with prepared salt and pepper, introduce in the oven at 400 degrees F and bake for 15 minutes.
- Season lamb with salt and pepper, place into a heated pan over medium high heat and cook for a couple of minutes.
- Add lamb to the baking dish with the fennel and figs, introduce in the oven and bake for 20 minutes more.
- Divide everything on plates and serve.
- Enjoy!

Nutritional Values: Calories 230; Carbs 5g; Fat 3g; Protein 10g

Pork Schnitzel

Serving Size: 4

Cooking Time: 20 minutes

Ingredients:

- 2-oz. flax seed, ground.
- 1-oz. sesame seed, ground.
- ½-cup milk.
- 1½-lbs. boneless pork loin slices.
- 2-tablespoon olive oil
- 2-tablespoon butter
- 2 eggs
- Pinch pepper and salt

Directions:

- Pound each pork slice until really thin. Mix the flaxseed, sesame, pepper and salt and spread out on a large plate
- Beat the prepared egg and milk together and season to taste. Coat the pork slices with egg and milk and then put them in the dry mixture. Make sure they are evenly coated.
- Place on a large plate covered with baking paper and rest in the fridge for 15 minutes. Heat the prepared oil and butter in a large non-stick skillet over a medium high heat
- Lay the pork slices in the oil and fry carefully until cooked and golden brown. About 4 minutes for each side.
- Drain on paper towel and serve whilst still hot. Serve with a crunchy green salad and lemon slices if liked.

Nutritional Values: Calories 486; Carbs 8.4g; Fat 30.3g; Protein 34.7g

Ricotta Cloud Pancakes with Whipped Cream

Serving Size: 4

Cooking Time: 10 minutes

Ingredients:

- 1 cup almond flour
- 1 teaspoon baking powder
- 2 ½ tablespoon swerve
- ⅓ teaspoon salt
- 1 ¼ cups ricotta cheese
- ⅓ cup coconut milk
- 2 large eggs
- 1 cup heavy whipping cream

Directions:

- In a large-sized bowl, whisk the almond flour, baking powder, swerve, and salt. Set aside.
- Crack the eggs into the blender and process on medium speed for 30 seconds. Add the ricotta cheese, continue processing it, and gradually pour the coconut milk in while you keep on blending. in about 90 seconds, the mixture will be creamy and smooth. Pour it into the dry ingredients and whisk to combine.
- Set a skillet over medium heat and let it heat for a minute. Then, fetch a soup spoonful of mixture into the skillet and cook it for 1 minute.
- Flip the pancake and cook further for 1 minute. Remove onto a plate and repeat the cooking process until the batter is exhausted. Serve the pancakes with whipping cream.

Nutritional Values: Calories 407; Carbs 6.6g; Fat 30.6g; Protein 11.5g

Sausage Egg Cups

Serving Size: 6

Cooking Time: 40 minutes

Ingredients:

- ½-lb. ground pork
- 12 large eggs
- 1 large avocado, peeled and diced.
- ¼-medium yellow onion, chopped.
- ¼-cup zucchini, chopped.
- Coconut oil to grease muffin tin.
- ½-teaspoon dried sage
- ¼-teaspoon red pepper flakes
- ½-teaspoon salt.
- ½-teaspoon black pepper

Directions:

- Preheat oven to a heat of 350 degrees F. Heat a large skillet over medium heat and add ground pork, sage, salt, black pepper and red pepper flakes. Cook until meat is no longer pink
- Now, remove pork mixture with a slotted spoon and set aside.
- Add onion and zucchini to pan and sauté until tender; about 4 minutes. Add cooked onion and zucchini to pork mixture in a medium bowl
- Add eggs to pork mixture and stir until combined. Oil each well of a 12-cup muffin tin with a small amount of coconut oil and pour mixture evenly into each well.
- Bake for 30 minutes or until egg is cooked through. Top each egg cup with a few pieces of avocado.

Nutritional Values: Calories 227; Carbs 3.5g; Fat 13.1g; Protein 20.3g

Shrimp and Olives Pan

Serving Size: 4

Cooking Time: 10 minutes

Ingredients:

- 1 pound shrimp, peeled and deveined
- 1 cup black olives, pitted and halved
- ½ cup kalamata olives, pitted and halved
- 2 spring onions, chopped
- 2 teaspoons sweet paprika
- 1 tablespoon olive oil
- Salt and black pepper to the taste
- ½ cup heavy cream

Directions:

- Heat up a large-sized pan with the oil over medium heat, add the onions, toss and cook for 2 minutes.
- Add the shrimp and the other ingredients except the cream, toss and cook for 4 minutes more.
- Add the cream, toss, cook over medium heat for another 4 minutes, divide everything between plates and serve for breakfast.

Nutritional Values: Calories 263; Carbs 5.5g; Fat 14.8g; Protein 26.7g

Shrimp Risotto

Serving Size: 4

Cooking Time: 15 minutes

Ingredients:

- 14 oz. shrimps, peeled and deveined
- 12 oz. cauli rice
- 4 button mushrooms
- ½ lemon
- 4 stalks green onion
- 3 tablespoon ghee butter
- 2 tablespoon coconut oil
- Salt and black pepper to taste

Directions:

- Preheat the oven to 400F
- Put a layer of cauli rice on a sheet pan, season with salt and spices; sprinkle the coconut oil over it
- Bake in the oven for 10-12 minutes
- Cut the green onion, slice up the mushrooms and remove the rind from the lemon
- Heat the ghee butter in a skillet over medium heat. Add the shrimps; season it and sauté for 5-6 minutes
- Top the cauli rice with the shrimps, sprinkle the green onion over it.

Nutritional Values: Calories 363; Carbs 9.2g; Fat 26.2g; Protein 25g

Veal Picatta

Serving Size: 2

Cooking Time: 15 minutes

Ingredients:

- 2 tablespoons ghee
- ¼ cup white wine
- ¼ cup chicken stock
- 1 and ½ tablespoons capers
- 1 garlic clove, minced
- 8 ounces veal scallops
- Salt and black pepper to the taste

Directions:

- Heat up a large-sized pan with half of the butter over medium high heat, add veal cutlets, season with salt and pepper, cook for 1 minute on each side and transfer to a plate.
- Heat up the large-sized pan again over medium heat, add garlic, stir and cook for 1 minute.
- Add wine, stir and simmer for 2 minutes.
- Add stock, capers, salt, pepper, the rest of the ghee and return veal to pan.
- Stir everything, cover pan and cook piccata on medium low heat until veal is tender.
- Enjoy!

Nutritional Values: Calories 204; Carbs 5g; Fat 12g; Protein 10g

Made in the USA
Las Vegas, NV
11 February 2023

67324597R00072